COVID SMART

A NURSE'S MEMOIR

ZENIA KAHAN

CONTENTS

To all the health care workers during the pandemic, and
especially the nurses and patient care workers who supported
me and each other on 5B.

Introduction

I've heard the saying: *May you live in interesting times.* It is a mixed blessing. COVID-19 brought tragedy and chaos while providing an opportunity for growth and progress. I never thought my career in nursing would end during a pandemic. Nurses deserve respect and increased compensation for the unprecedented challenges thrown at us. We also deserved respect before the pandemic. The virus is still with us, and we still need to assess the ongoing risk of spreading it.

When a new pandemic emerged, it came in waves. So many waves, we stopped counting. Unlike Japan's iconic *The Great Wave* (depicted by the artist Hokusai, 1831), these waves were not only focused on the nearest shore. The COVID-19 waves spread far and wide around the world. It was like an invisible tsunami until the development and distribution of vaccines. But then, the waves continued with variants of the original virus. This virus would mutate again and again and again.

How deadly this virus became depended mostly on the pattern of human behaviour. How each country responded was determined by their politicians and the willingness of citizens to care more for their fellow human beings than their own presumed inalienable freedoms or accustomed lifestyles.

Canada showed it cared and prioritized responses for the elderly, the sick, and the vulnerable. However, the pandemic also revealed cracks in every country's health care system and culture, including our own. In Canada, each province and territory have the responsibility to provide health care. They manage poorly at times because of political priorities and interference, lack of funding, shortage of health care staff, limited access [to health care due to the distance between communities] and/or other reasons.

It is shameful that Ontario, the largest province, claims it needs more federal money for health care. Premier Doug Ford and his Conservative provincial government wasted taxpayers' money on stickers to rebel against federal gasoline taxes. They also squandered money on ineffective blue provincial licence plates (that cannot be read at a distance) but have not fixed the problem. Then they gave away money, when they discontinued licence plate renewal fees and gave refunds for the last two years of paid renewals. The latest act of hypocrisy is the reduction of provincial sales taxes on gas, while complaining about the federal tax, which they want access to. No wonder Ford's government has less money (and less respect) for health care or health care workers—especially our nurses.

Before the pandemic, Premier Ford and his government decided the best way to reduce the provincial debt was to reduce their largest expenditure—provincial public servants' salaries. It was simple arithmetic for them. And so, Bill 124 was born. No consideration for whom this affected or the consequences of this very bad decision. It's as if nurses were **nonessential** health care workers instead of essential ones.

The Ontario Nurses' Association (ONA) is one of the unions that took immediate action to repeal Bill 124. Other unions joined the fight and repealed this wage suppression bill successfully three years later. However, instead of initiating reparations, the provincial government is appealing the court's decision. No respect for the court, or for nurses.

During the 5th COVID-19 wave the far-right convoy protests emerged. Chaos, frustration, and anger reached a crescendo as the Ontario provincial government failed to act for fear of losing their majority status in the next election. Therefore, the federal government had to step in with the Emergencies Act to protect Canada's economic security, international reputation, and sovereignty.

Walk the 100,000 steps (both mental and physical) of nurses as they do their daily professional care. See how the work became more intense during this pandemic. Feel the shock of how Canadian news affected those still fighting the good fight. And then, know that nurses are worthy of your respect.

PART I

WHAT NURSES DO

CHAPTER 1

Nurses are Professionals

I had a vague idea of what nurses did. I was so wrong. Unless you are in the nursing profession or work closely with hospital nurses, you have no idea how hard they work. And neither did I before I became a nurse. Television and films rarely depict the challenging work and impossible circumstances that drag nurses into prioritizing their daily tasks. Consequently, these factors result in conflicting emotions and depressing spirits. This is my account of bedside nursing during the first two years of the COVID-19 pandemic.

But first, what are registered nurses? They are professional, essential health care workers, who have a Bachelor of Science degree in Nursing or a grandfathered equivalent nursing diploma. Before 2005 it used to be a Diploma of Nursing for all entry-level nurses in Ontario. Someone thought the degree program would elevate nurses' standing in the community or with employers. Sadly, it did not.

Respect is earned, or is it? Despite courses in anatomy, physiology, health assessment, pharmacotherapeutics, epidemiology, research, psychology, ethics, leadership, and various clinical rotations, nurses still do not have the respect or similar consideration of other professionals. This is reflected by nurses' union contracts continuously decided by arbitration. Most recently Ontario's Bill 124 (2019) has limited nurses' wage increases by 1% per year, while doctors' union contracts are settled by negotiation with an ambiguous year-three raise (March 2022). It doesn't sound like 1% each year to me. Perhaps respect is subjective and not earned.

Alas, only the College of Nurses of Ontario (CNO) seems to recognize the earned nursing degree. The College is the gatekeeper of who can practise nursing in their jurisdiction, based on entry to practice requirements, current work status, and any public practice complaints. Their *Find a Nurse* website also allows the public to make complaints more easily. As such, this respect is temporary and fragile, at best.

Although, to be fair, the CNO only protects the public, and is the rhetoric I've always heard from other nurses. Doctors also have a comparable website, which includes their medical education. I can see the need for the public to check out a doctor prior to their initial appointment in a non-hospital setting. However, nurses in hospitals are assigned to patients, and there's no time or real need to verify their credentials. It's already been done by their employer when hired.

There is no oath in Ontario for nurses like the doctors' Hippocratic Oath. However, nurses know they cannot talk about their patients beyond the circle of care. Confidentiality is one of the principles of nursing. Yet, I had to sign a privacy form as part of my eLearning courses. It was a no-brainer that I couldn't talk about my patients, but maybe I shouldn't talk about or, at least, reveal the name of my hospital too.

Therefore, based on the two annual privacy forms and the hospital forum talks, I decided not to name my employer or my hospital. After all, I wanted to describe a Toronto acute care hospital bedside nurse's COVID-19 experience. The emphasis should be on my lived experience, and not on which hospital I worked at.

Nurses learn their craft on the job. The actual practical work of hospital nurses happens at the bedside. Orientation with a buddy nurse is never enough. Then it becomes independent learning. The clinical educator and

Charge Nurse can only be a stop gap measure. Learn by doing. Experience will always matter. Knowledge, skills, and ability are the nurse's professional standard. And being able to react to changes in a patient's condition is crucial. Comforting families without stealing time from other patients is an art and another big challenge.

No one truly prepares nurses on how to balance their care and patients' needs with that of doctors, allied health (like physio or occupational therapists), and porters, who need to take patients for tests or procedures. Orientation on the job only gives a taste of what's ahead. One thing is clear. Nurses have limited time, resources, and energy, as well as other deserving or "demanding" patients and their family members.

The nurse-patient relationship is supposed to be therapeutic. The College states this relationship is composed of trust, respect, professional intimacy, empathy, and power. I rarely felt any power over my patients, mainly because nurses are true givers —caregivers. They have a primary duty of care to the patient, which can seem difficult at times to balance against other needs or requirements. Hence, they earn their respect every minute on the job.

CHAPTER 2

A Sign from the Universe

As previously mentioned, I wasn't aware of what nurses did when I got into nursing in 2000. I knew of nurses on soap operas like *General Hospital*, and dramas like *ER*. I didn't know about the nationwide nurses' shortages of 20,000 or the nurse layoffs of the 1990s in Ontario. This was not in the headlines of the daily news that I read or heard.

Nursing was the furthest thing from my mind when graduating from high school. I thought nursing was too feminine and passive, and that doctors ordered nurses around.

My father ordered me around already. There were many expectations of me: I had to do household chores, go to Ukrainian school after regular school, as well as Ukrainian scouts (Plast) meetings, attend church every Sunday, and obey my parents even when I disagreed. I wanted something with power, or at least equal power.

My father was the boss of everyone in the family and he expected obedience. There was little negotiation for outside interests. He held the purse strings and there were no allowances in this family. I also had no money until I found part-time jobs as a teenager. Since I was the youngest, I also never saw or knew how my other siblings dealt with this. Although, my two brothers did move out as soon as they could.

My immediate need was to move out of my parents' home too. I grew up in a Ukrainian-Canadian family (my parents were first-generation immigrants) in Toronto. We had a boarding house in Chinatown, which we continued to rent out once we moved to Bloor West Village. I resented this move as a 5-year-old, because we still didn't have discretionary money for candy and later, for new clothes.

I wasn't an only child. My parents had five children in total. Two sons, then two daughters, then I arrived years after the death of Lesia in 1959, who was the first daughter. By all accounts, Lesia was a happy and good-natured child. She got along with everyone. She also received a lot of candy for her angelic behaviour.

Lesia had a sweet tooth. Her downfall was that candy. She was 5 years old when she died 18 hours after visiting the dentist for an infected tooth. In those days, people were sedated by gas, instead of freezing by injection. A wellness call was made the following day, ironically, before she died while watching tv. Her heart just stopped. CPR wasn't invented until 1960.

The coroner's jury ruled death due to unknown causes. After " the most intensive postmortem study was conducted … nothing to indicate what caused her death" (The Globe and Mail, August 27, 1959). I only discovered this follow-up article recently. And I find this decision inconceivable and unacceptable by today's standards.

We became a family with four children again, once I was born. I may not have known this sister, but her death permeated our family dynamics, and affected my world view. My family rarely spoke of her. It was like some dark family secret.

However, this was an unbearable loss for my mother. My mother would speak of Lesia whenever I misbehaved. She would compare us. I felt like the black sheep of the family. I tried hard to make up for not being the angel she had lost.

It was because of this conflict of trying to appease my mother and rebelling against my father's rules that I needed my own independence and freedom. The first step was to leave my parents' home. I found an apartment to rent within six months of obtaining a full-time job.

On the last day of high school, I skipped school to fill out job applications at major employers like banks. CIBC Mortgage Life Insurance offered me a clerical job. This allowed me to move several months later to a flat in a house on Macdonell Avenue. I thought I'd only stay a year at CIBC, but this turned out to be 12 years.

My banking career was going nowhere. I saw having a degree meant promotions to higher paying jobs. They didn't pay me well, and I lived paycheck to paycheck. I couldn't even afford to contribute to my company pension. Then, when we finally had a union, they squashed it the next year.

In the following years my working life did not improve. Then, in 1993, the company decided to reorganize. That was a bad situation for everyone I knew. I already had plans to quit in 1992, but the federal government announced changes to Unemployment Insurance (UI), now known as Employment Insurance, which would disqualify me. Fate was kind later when my job became redundant, and I would be eligible for benefits.

Instead of reapplying for my old position, I left to finish my part-time BA degree at York University. I still didn't know what I wanted to do. I was interested in the environmental movement. So, I ended up with an Environmental Studies bachelor's degree, and no job prospects. The job market had changed.

I was getting desperate. I had applied to so many jobs, both part-time and full-time. I had kept a list just in case UI asked. My list recorded 40 employment opportunities for which I didn't even get a call back. My degree was meaningless. I was already in my thirties, but I couldn't even get a casual coffee shop job in my neighbourhood. They now wanted young, experienced "baristas," or so I was told. As a teenager I had no problem getting jobs. Now I was the outsider.

I even tried to become a police officer, but didn't pass the interview. I had bought my first car several years before and probably didn't pass a background credit check. Or maybe it was the fact I had moved so many times for various reasons. I wasn't told. I should have asked my neighbour, a police sergeant, for help, but I was too embarrassed and too proud. I wanted to get a job on my own like I did as a teenager.

One thing that kept me going and grounded was my interest in all things spiritual and healing. I may have tried to contact my deceased sister with a Ouija board. I did dabble in the paranormal, transcendental meditation, and spiritual healing arts. I even took courses at the Spiritual Science Institute of Canada in 1989. Then, in the 1990s, I got fully involved in the Reiki (hands on) and Therapeutic Touch (hands off) energy healing movements. I was advised providing two modalities of healing would make me more successful as a practitioner.

Reiki is a Japanese healing modality based on the teachings of Dr. Mikao Usui in the late 1880s. It uses the unlimited potential of the "universal life energy" to focus this healing energy into the energy systems of the client. Reiki treats the whole person on all levels: physical, mental, emotional, and spiritual. Most practitioners use a massage table for the comfort of the client (and practitioner) and access to all body locations. There are ten formal hand positions on the body, but some practitioners are "called" to additional areas.

This felt like a vocation for me. I felt like a sponge for healing knowledge and was intent on service to others. I took both levels and then audited them with other teachers. Much later in 2012 I would return to Reiki teachings and go to Glastonbury, UK to do my Master Level. It was quite the experience, surrounded by local King Arthur legends and New Age shops.

On the other hand, Therapeutic Touch (TT) is a healing system developed by Americans Dolores Krieger and Dora Kunz. Here, the object was to sense the person's aura (the electro-magnetic field) and help balance it with sweeping hand motions in the aura. The client could be on a chair or a massage table.

The Therapeutic Touch Network (TTN) protected this evidence-based healing art with case studies, and more rigid rules for what defines TT. It attracted many nurses, as Dolores was an RN herself. While I attended TTN meetings in Toronto, I also went with my friend to one of their retreats at Pumpkin Hollow, in Craryville, NY. There, I met Dora Kunz, who excelled at reading auras and had published several books on the topic. It was a real privilege.

However, I resonated best with Reiki and tried to make a living as a holistic health practitioner. In December 1996 I had a stall for Reiki at the Whole Life Expo at the Metro Toronto Convention Centre. Then I followed up with local talks in January and April 1997, a weekly TT clinic at the Swansea Town Hall, and rented space for Reiki on Dundas St. West near Bloor St. West. I believed I was finally on my way to financial independence.

That didn't happen. My business was very slow, and I was always ambivalent about charging clients for Reiki. Good thing I was living with my parents again. But I worried that my eldest brother would talk my father into kicking me out at some point. I was very anxious every time he visited. He had my father's ear. So, I kept myself scarce when I heard his voice in the house. I just needed more time to figure out my situation.

After a while, I discovered a pattern of clients asking about their "occipital" or other body parts during a Reiki session. There was no Internet or personal computers during this time. I guess I could've gone to the library and checked a dictionary. But I was curious too. So, I ended up taking a course in anatomy at Humber College. And I did exceptionally well.

Students continuously asked if I was in the Nursing Program. It was ridiculous how often I got asked. I eventually realized this was a sign from the universe. I reckoned nursing would be a steady income. That turned out to be true. I enrolled in the nursing program in the winter semester of 2000.

In 2001, when 9/11 happened, I was at school. I had just finished a class at 10:00 a.m. and was exiting the room. Everyone was standing about in groups and were unnaturally quiet in the hallways. I heard murmurs about something in the student lounge, and so I went there. On the TV screens hanging from the ceilings were repeated video images of planes crashing into buildings in New York City (NYC). I didn't hear any newscasters' commentary. They must have been in shock and speechless. Why a second plane? Why NYC? Anti-capitalists? Why not Washington, DC, which would be an obvious military target? I didn't hear about United Airlines Flight 93 enroute to Washington or the attack on the Pentagon until much later.

Humber College's North Campus lies beneath the flightpath towards the Toronto Pearson International Airport. I was used to seeing airplanes flying overhead every few minutes. It was eerie how empty and silent the skies were that day.

While I was waiting for the bus, I saw a classmate freaking out. She said her cousin worked in one of the towers that was hit. He must be dead. Her friends couldn't console her. When I saw her next, she was unusually quiet. I never asked if she truly lost her cousin that day. It felt impolite.

In the beginning, I naively believed I could combine Reiki and nursing. I thought I would have time to do energy healing when I started working as a nurse. It would be a win-win situation for me. There had to be time for this. If there ever was, then I was too busy, too tired, or not grounded enough to be of any help in that way. However, this is how I got into nursing.

CHAPTER 3

A Double-Minted Nurse

I applied to several Toronto hospitals as a new nursing graduate in 2002. The first one quizzed me on different types of shock. I failed that interview as I didn't recall that fever accompanies septic shock. In fact, I said, "it couldn't be shock." The next hospital only offered me a part-time job. I wouldn't get any hands-on experience at that rate. I wanted a full-time job with a steady income.

The third hospital took me because they remembered me from my clinical rotation the previous year. No quizzes. This time I was given refreshments. However, this full-time position was for a nurse in a resource pool between three units. I never knew where I'd be until one of the three units claimed me for the day. It wasn't a perfect fit, but I would have a steady income.

It was scary. My lack of real nursing experience haunted me. None of the staff nurses seemed approachable or offered to help me. But they were busy too. Each unit was slightly different. Spinal, neurosurgery, and neurology had different layouts, but the nursing cultures in each one was generally unfriendly. Even the patient care assistants (PCAs) would help their favourite nurse first. I despaired about finding any real help.

After a year, I recognized the approachable nurses and applied to their unit once a position opened. But when I got there those nice nurses were not on my rotation, so I had to rely heavily on the Charge Nurse and the clinical educators. The Charge Nurse was soon tired of me.

Not all Charge Nurses are created equal. Some are less helpful. I think it comes down to your personality and your beliefs about what nursing is or should be. The more you care about your patients, the more you will advocate on their behalf. I got attached to my patients and couldn't let go of worrying about their progress. Maybe that's what made me a good Charge Nurse despite my dread and stress of being chosen. I always felt like a target, having to defend attacks or comply with requests from all directions: other nurses, doctors, patients, and family members. It was lonely, too.

The phrase, it's lonely at the top, can apply here. No one wanted the additional stress of being the Charge Nurse. My best work friend was the usual Charge Nurse, but I was selected frequently when she was on vacation or absent. I was not comfortable making decisions on the spot. I preferred advanced planning and thoughtful decision-making. Instead, I felt like I was always protecting my centre of gravity (energetically grounded) all the time from others' requests, demands, or complaints.

My earlier lack of specific nursing experience made me anxious, but I reached out to clinical educators. Some of the former ones told me to look up my answers in the hospital's clinical policies. It took years to find an understanding clinical educator (who wanted to teach) and for the other nurses to warm up to me. I guess, by then, I wasn't the new nurse anymore.

In the meantime, I went back to school part-time for a nursing degree at Ryerson University (now known as Toronto Metropolitan University). I didn't want the new nursing graduates to know more than me. They didn't. It was just more academic education, on how to read research papers, and write essays or articles. However, I felt more confident because I was now a "double-minted" registered nurse (RN), and I had more hospital experience under my belt. I should have been worth my weight in gold. Instead, I received a temporary small stipend for a year for upgrading my credentials.

When it came time for me to be a pre-graduate student's preceptor, I was ready. The first few students were enthusiastic and willing to learn. I really did not feel much of a generational gap until later. Each school program had different ways of assessing the student's progress, so I had to adjust as well, completing more online evaluations as opposed to writing comments on a form.

Then I had students who were not inclined to do the work at all. I was flabbergasted they had gotten so far into the program. For one student, it was her last chance to get a degree, after other educational misadventures. Another one planned to create a website for nursing students, which I thought was very ambitious, and failed to produce it by the end of term. His school gave him a make-up project, unheard of in my time.

Working with students was more work at the bedside. Everything took longer to explain, supervise, and evaluate. Some nurses thought I should get a heavier assignment because there were two of us (the student and me). However, a student is not equal to a registered nurse. Far from it. I felt like I was walking with a puppy attached to my foot.

Then I came upon a diamond. This student shone and made working life a joy. She followed instructions, clarified why we were doing things, was pleasant, but most of all, she was reliable. She was the only one I recommended we hire right away. Instead, she chose the unit next to us.

Not all staff nurses were assigned "pre-grad" students. I was told this was part of my duties as a full-time nurse. I didn't notice at first who else had students, but over time only a few of us did. We did get a small supplement for the extra responsibility. Teaching the next generation of nurses felt like passing on the torch. So, I was disappointed more people weren't involved. These other nurses had valuable skills that needed sharing.

CHAPTER 4

A Day in the Life of a Nurse

How does a typical day in my hospital unit look? I have been on the same unit for about 18 years, but it has not been boring or predictable. This part of my memoir is not meant to be a handbook for new nurses, but rather, proof of the hard mental, emotional, and physical work of hospital nurses who are worthy of more than a 1% wage increase.

To begin, my unit had "stable" patients from neurology, neurosurgery, and an epilepsy specialty mini unit. Neurology patients were looking for a diagnosis or treatment. Their conditions ran the gamut of multiple sclerosis, Parkinson's Disease (PD), Stiff Person Syndrome, seizures, and dementias. Neurosurgery patients usually had brain cancer, benign growths, traumatic subdural hemorrhages, trigeminal neuralgia, or plans for implantation of a deep brain stimulation (mostly for PD). There were a lot of crossovers between the neurology, neurosurgery, and epilepsy services for diagnosing and treating epilepsy in patients.

The 12-hour nursing day shift starts with getting your patient assignment of four patients. The Charge Nurse noted these in the assignment book the previous day. So, if staff called in sick just hours before the shift, then there wouldn't be enough time to replace the sick nurse and the remaining day staff may get five patients instead. Or maybe the manager doesn't allow the first sick call to be replaced for budgetary reasons. The nursing pool was usually in high demand. Therefore, the start of your workday was unpredictable.

Nurses pick up a copy of the unit's census of patients for reference as well as to write their notes about their patients. I would use the back of the sheet and fold it into eights (to have extra space for a fifth patient or extra tasks). Then they move on to the nursing plan (known as the Kardex) for each patient, which is found in several binders.

The Kardex describes the patient's admitting diagnosis, medical history, recent surgery, and doctors' orders. Orders may include frequency of vital signs (VS) and neurological (neuro) assessments, oxygen minimum requirements, existing stomas (e.g., tracheostomy, colostomy) or nasogastric tubes, IV sites, POCT frequency (point-of-care testing for glucose), urinary catheters, and diet. Nurses also add important "need-to-know" things like the last bowel movement (LBM), height, weight, family contact, or expected plans like discharge disposition.

LBM is very important for surgical patients. During surgery the GI system slows down. After surgery nurses will follow up and may order a bowel routine (medications) to move the bowels and tell the patient to get up and walk. Best practice is early mobilization post-op for lungs and bowels.

Ileus (temporary loss of intestinal peristalsis) is a serious post-op condition, which can lead to necrosis (tissue death) and peritonitis (inflammation of the inner wall of the abdomen). Once you see someone vomit feces, it's "game over," unless emergency surgery happens fast enough. Obstructed bowels are not good, either. Neurosurgeons are primarily concerned about your brain. Nurses are concerned about your whole body, and this is why they auscultate your abdomen for bowel sounds.

After the Kardex, nurses must check the computer for their patients' medications and their due times, bloodwork, other tests, and/or results. Also, the night shift nurses try to give verbal reports to the day shift as soon as possible. If time permits, nurses pull out the morning meds before visiting their patients. All this before the morning Charge Report at 7:45 in the Charting Room. The day shift officially starts at 7:30. Is it any wonder I would come in early? I would aim for 6:30.

For many years I would come early, but the night shift didn't like this. Some nurses would keep the patient's Kardex page throughout the shift. So, I would have to hunt this down. In recent years I have seen more nurses come early too. This is unpaid time, but it helps with reducing stress.

Bedside reporting is considered nursing best practice. Nurses are to give updates on patients in front of the patients. Theoretically, transparency of information is desirable. Nurses can also quickly check if their patients are still sleeping in bed (haven't fallen going to the bathroom) and have the expected equipment or devices, as well as whether IV bags are still full and urinary bags need to be drained. Nurses are also expected to update the patient's whiteboard with their name, the current date, and any outstanding tests or procedures.

Once upon a time, we made taped reports for our patients. I was so bad at it, too many "ums" and "ahs" that my manager gave me a cassette recording of my report. How embarrassing! Later, reporting was written on a preformatted sheet. However, I believe the best reporting is verbal with the oncoming nurse. There's no limit to content and this allows for warnings on potential problems or challenges.

However, this bedside reporting is problematic. If the patient is asleep, having two nurses talking may wake them up. Patients don't mind if doctors wake them, but not if it's the nurses. Also, on our unit, up to a third are confused, so including them in the bedside report may cause agitation. Then there are patients who are challenging at the best of times. No one wants to start their day alienating their patients. This antagonizes the necessary therapeutic nurse-patient relationship that nurses need to be effective and affective.

There is also the problem of timing for the previous shift nurses. They may still be charting or doing things for their patients. We have until 15 minutes past shift change to give reports on the patients to each nurse. It's not just one nurse giving a report to another. One might have to get reports from several nurses. Assignments change. A patient's status may change.

This is another reason I came early to work. I needed a moment to reset and accept my assignment and refocus.

The day shift is a marathon of activities, but nurses don't get to choose their pace. The best laid plans can get thrown out the window fast. After the Charge Report is done it's a sprint to get the vital signs (VS) machines, then get the VS and neuro assessments done before the medications are due. Our nurses are expected to use mobile computers that have drawers for the medications that lock. Funny how these drawers worked for several months before they started getting stuck. User friendly?

These computers also found wireless dead zones in hallways or in patients' rooms. This was frustrating and embarrassing. For this reason, I always preferred reliable desktop computers. These wireless (computers) on wheels (WOWs) were more like the COWs (computers on wheels) they were originally named for. Sometimes it is hard to move or use. I'm from the city, but maybe rural nurses feel differently about calling the computers cows. I know in Britain "cow" has been used as a negative slang about girls or women. So, WOW is more politically correct.

Patient call bells are another technology that is usually a good thing. They work better than the WOWs, because they rely on electricity. They allow patients to call for assistance getting out of bed, being changed, reminding nurses of their missed or forgotten pain medications, or for some other reason.

I've heard of "call bell retraining," at a nursing symposium, for patients who misused the call bell system. I have never seen anyone successfully retrained. On our unit some patients are very confused or perhaps not fluent enough in English and may not understand that the call bell is not a toy. Also, the call bell must be cleared at the bedside to turn off the call light in front of the patient's room.

I remember one patient who called because she was lonely. She was a young woman in a private room. I got frustrated very quickly, but she was a fall risk and so I needed to check on her every time. I had her as a patient several times before I came up with the idea of playing the song "[It Isn't] In My Blood" by Shawn Mendes. I would sing along to the first line, "Help me, [help me] it's like the walls are caving in," and play the music video on my cell for us. (I paraphrased his song title because the repeating phrase is longer and means the opposite).

I realized this was not professional at all, but once I did it, I really enjoyed it. I think she did too. It let me continue to respond to her calls without getting angry, calming us both down. Who doesn't like Shawn's music?

Family members use the call bell as well for the patient's peri-care (perineal-care) needs (e.g., assisting/transferring via commode chair to the washroom or changing adult diapers), updates from nurses, or just trying to reach the doctor. Nurses are not the gatekeepers to access the doctor. Even the Charge Nurse at the Nurses' Station can only page doctors under certain circumstances.

The call bell rings directly to the nurse assigned to the patient. Nurses carry pager-like devices that notify which bed is calling. Some people call it a cellphone with limited features. These pagers are an improvement over the overhead call systems, which made the unit quite a bit noisier than it had to be.

Sometimes the unit clerk would transfer phone calls to the nurse without notice. These calls could be from the MRI (magnetic resonance imaging) or CT (computer tomography) department asking questions about the nurse's patient. At other times it's the family member asking questions. The sound quality is not always perfect. It may be due to the wireless dead zones again.

Unfortunately, I have given the wrong update at least once or twice. That's why I got upset when this happened. Then I had to investigate who really had called and apologize. These pagers did not have a call display. I much preferred answering family enquiries from a desk phone at the Nurses' Station (when I wasn't attending to a patient).

I remember a time when technology promised to make work life easier. It has become another tool to provide more access to information, whether we need it or not.

CHAPTER 5

Patient-Centred Care Challenges

Technology was but one of the obstacles to time management. Some patients preferred medications with their meals. Nurses may have to return to them later if that was the case. We are not supposed to leave medications at the bedside. Remember, nurses are to witness medication swallowing, but also need to build and maintain a therapeutic relationship with their patients.

At times, this made me feel more like a servant (or a personal maid) than a nurse. Doing customer service instead of professional nursing care. In the nursing diploma program, we explored various nursing care models. Patient-centred care was the popular hospital model to provide best health outcomes and patient satisfaction. Somehow, the idealized patient-centred care (or circle of care model) became the patient (and/or family) is always right. No wonder in school they kept calling patients clients. They meant customers, as with the American health care system.

My mantra would be "smile and try to move on," or "keep calm and carry on" like the British saying on my staff lounge cup. I tried to focus on getting things done as my list of duties and tasks was long.

Nurses had to make sure meals were delivered to all their patients. Some patients needed to be fed. Others complained about the food and their food allergies, sensitivities, or dislikes. If that's the case, then nurses must review their patient's diet orders and see if anything needs to be updated. And if it's beyond the nurse, then the kitchen technician gets called in. The dietitian is mostly limited to dealing with enteral feeds (nutrition for NG or G-tubes) on our unit. The dietitian does not deal with preferences. My hospital does not provide options like keto diets. Nurses keep having to explain this repeatedly.

Every meal is a potential crisis for the food sensitive patient. This can appear unreasonable to a busy nurse. I felt sometimes like a waitress (without the restaurant kitchen). I would remind patients they were allowed to bring in their own food or order in. One patient left the hospital because we couldn't accommodate his "allergy" to processed food. We do manage to adapt for several items like MSG, but it can greatly reduce the food options. Meanwhile, a small percentage of patients loved the hospital food. Go figure!

Obviously, patients should be sitting upright for meals. For patients with enteral feeds their head of bed (HOB) should be elevated at minimum to 30 degrees to prevent nausea or reflux.

For post-op surgical patients this same rule applies while in hospital, but to prevent facial edema, which means swelling of the face (especially around the eyes) and for any neurosurgical drains to work. It's still hard for me to watch TV medical patients lying flat in bed while on oxygen. Sitting up helps to expand the lungs.

At some point during this busy period, nurses are expected to chart about their patients in a *timely manner*. Nurses must confirm they received the shift report, and document in what condition they found their patients, any new or ongoing issues, and if any follow-up was done. I'm lucky if I can write something by 11:00 a.m., but not lucky if an issue arises.

These are some examples that should interrupt the nurse's workflow. If the patient has a temperature of 38.5 degrees Celsius, then the Charge Nurse needs to call the doctor for a febrile work-up, and the nurse follows the orders for the patient. Another situation would be excessive bleeding after surgery. Nurses must show they made assessments and if a notable change is observed, then action is required.

For the nurse, this means reporting it and for the doctor, remedying it with orders or coming to the unit to insert additional sutures.

Additionally, if a stable patient becomes unstable, then the nurse must document this as soon as possible after taking vitals, neuro assessments and any other actions to keep the patient safe while asking the Charge Nurse to call the doctor. It's not always the doctor who is called. Depending on the service or circumstances, it may be a nurse practitioner (NP), or a medical protocol like Code Blue. The usual stat orders are for bloodwork, IV insertion of a saline lock (if no IV access), IV bolus or medication, or a CT scan.

Lawyers tell nurses that if it wasn't charted, it didn't happen. If not charted, then a poorer second defence (or evidence) is the nurse's usual practice. Nurses worry about losing their nursing licence. Some nurses worry so much about this that they double document (in the chart and online) vitals and other assessments.

When I started nursing in 2002, I was told online charting was coming to our hospital soon. Instead, we used paper charts, which had to be shared by other team members. It was frustrating not to have access to the chart when the doctor or therapists were using it. There's a lot to remember while busy moving on to the next task. I know that at Humber River Hospital they already had online charting, but their nurses only had access to one desktop computer on their unit. That was during my first clinical rotation as a student.

In June 2022, compete online charting became the new standard at my hospital. No more paper charts. Previously I was told to document in the narrative style in the chart. Later we had switched to tick marks on forms and charting by exception, but now it's all online.

With the new online charting, we didn't immediately realize that we would also be scanning barcodes for practically everything a nurse enters online, and the medications or blood products given to patients. I don't know if this will eventually make things easier for nurses, or worse. The skeptic in me says the scanning of barcode products is to keep track of inventory, and that safety is a secondary goal.

I recall early in my career a nurse who left because we were transitioning from paper medication records to online medication orders. I was excited about this, but she saw it as one too many changes for her. I guess I am in her shoes now and can sympathize with her decision.

The learning curve is expected to be very steep, and I sincerely hope the wireless computers are more reliable this time. I fear the nurses will spend more time with these computers and scanners than with the patient. I hope I'm wrong.

CHAPTER 6

Hygiene and Wound Care

One of the basics of nursing is keeping the patient clean and dry. Good hygiene helps the patient to feel good and recover or heal. Therefore, a patient can call a nurse at any time to be changed from a soiled diaper (but not at shift change). When I began in 2002, we had two PCAs on day shift and one on nights. Their shift began 30 minutes before the new nurses arrived. They would cover the patients' calls during shift change.

The staffing formula has changed over the years, and now in 2022, we have one PCA on day shift and on evenings only. However, my unit has patients with moderate to severe weaknesses. It takes two staff members to lift, slide, and turn patients after a diaper change.

We also had registered practical nurses (RPNs) who used to share patients with the RNs. They would do hygiene care, but not medication. Their scope of practice changed to include medication and we lost our RPNs (they didn't want to upgrade their skills). In recent years, we have RPNs again, but now they have complete responsibility for their patients, and they must be stable. Therefore, replacing one RPN for one RN per shift saves money. It also means that the RN's patient load is heavier than before.

Two staff members to change a total-care patient is best practice. Injuries can happen to the nurse, PCA, or the patient during this manoeuvre. The nurse uses the call bell system for assistance. Sometimes everyone is busy or maybe the nurse or patient can't wait. I have suffered chronic tendonitis from this in the past. But it's still hard to walk away and not help immediately. If you are lucky, it's close to nursing rounds time.

Nursing rounds are nothing like doctors' rounds, where a team of doctors see their patients once a day. Nursing rounds happen at 2:00 p.m., 1:00 a.m., and 5:00 a.m. This is when all available nurses (and the PCA, at 2:00 p.m.) check on all the patients and, if necessary, change diapers; lift patients up in bed (they always slide down to the foot of the bed), then turn them on a new side; or transfer patients to wheelchairs. The Charge Nurse and PCA do additional hygiene rounds at 4:00 p.m. and 9:00 p.m. Nurses are always busy.

Morning or "a.m. care" is usually done before lunch. Part of organizing one's patient assignment is to know who needs a bed bath, and who just needs washing supplies. Generally, if a patient can walk and has no weakness in their arms or hands, supplies should be enough, unless they ask for a shower. Then the nurse must check if the shower room is clean, safe, and unoccupied. There are only two shower rooms, excluding the private rooms.

I am forever grateful for the PCA who takes my complete-care patient to the shower. It's the only way to wash hair properly. As the nurse, I don't feel I have time for this. I do have the 5–10 minutes to assist the PCA with the ceiling lift to position the patient into or out of the shower chair.

Bed baths are more efficient timewise for the nurse. Supplies are brought to the bedside; curtains are closed for privacy; feed pump is turned off, if applicable; the bed is flattened and raised to the nurse's hip level; the patient's skin is assessed during the wash from head/face to toe and dried; and a new hospital gown and diaper is put on. Assistance for a quick boost up in bed is called. Then oral care can be done at this time.

I miss the days when visiting hours started at 11:00 and the nurses and PCAs had a chance to make the patients clean and presentable for their families. However, maybe families need to have firsthand knowledge of what is involved. A behind-the-curtains reality check of the challenges faced by nurses.

•••

Meanwhile, all hospital nurses should aspire to continuously improve their wound care. Everyone should know the skin is the largest external organ and the first layer of protection against infection and injury. I'm very concerned about the quality of my patient's skin as I used to suffer from acne. I think that's why I found myself passionate about patient wound care. Everyone values healthy looking skin that is clear and unblemished, or a pale scar from a healed surgical incision.

The easy wounds are surgical. For neurosurgical patients we have a unit protocol for the first four days after surgery. It used to be that each surgeon would have a stated preference for when dressings should be removed or when hair could be washed.

In the last decade a protocol developed for consistency. The nurse can now remove the turban or strip dressing after post-op day two. Of course, if there's a Jackson Pratt™ (JP) drain attached, this may delay things. Once the drain is removed, a new suture is added. Most craniotomies have surgical staples that close the incision. A redo craniotomy has sutures for better healing.

Part of wound care involves assessment of the wound, and cleaning and applying a new dressing—usually a Medipore™ strip dressing. This is repeated on post-op day three.

However, on post-op day four the dressing is removed and kept off (open to air) unless there's a concern. Some patients may have increased swelling, redness, or oozing of blood. If so, this is reported to the doctor upon first discovery. Otherwise, if everything looks good, the nurse will continue to clean the wound. All wound assessments and treatments are documented.

I remember being disturbed by a relatively new nurse who sent a patient home with the original OR dressing. He did not even "look under the hood." There were dried blood stains on the dressing. I was embarrassed that my colleague was so unprofessional and uncaring. Would he do this to his father? His excuse was he wasn't told about the dressing protocol.

Whenever a patient had a different kind of wound, I would be called. Not because I'm an expert, but my nurses knew I truly wanted to see and understand what could be done.

Wound care is within the nurse's scope of practice. Plastics is a separate medical service that deals with facial or scalp grafts. We don't get doctors' orders for chronic pressure wounds. Instead, we would call the Wound Care nurse to assess and write orders.

Cutbacks to hospital care over the years have reduced staff to the Wound Care team and lost the lone floating Diabetic Education nurse. If wound prevention is cheaper than treatment, then patients who are newly diagnosed diabetics need this early intervention. Diabetic pressure wounds take longer to heal.

In the last few years nurses at my hospital were "promoted" to be able to assess and treat Stage Two pressure wounds on their own. These are shallow wounds with broken skin. Stage One are wounds with consistent redness, but intact skin. These can be monitored or cushioned with a dressing like Mepilex®. If on the heels, then hospital "booties" can be used.

Pressure wounds or ulcers (in the hospital) are wounds that develop from being in one body position too long. All immobile patients are expected to be turned every two to four hours. I think I managed only twice in a 12-hour shift: during the a.m. bed bath and afternoon rounds. Some patients with very frail skin might get a specialty mattress. Turning patients every two hours was impossible when there were so many other priorities.

Some people are more prone to these wounds. My mother had an unstageable pressure wound from sitting in her customized wheelchair at the nursing home. The wound was on her ischium. This bone is known as "the sitting bone." I knew she'd return to bed after lunch for a nap, then go back to the wheelchair for several hours.

In contrast, in my hospital the Wound Care nurse would debride the necrotic tissue either by using a scalpel or debriding cream. In the nursing home a Home Care nurse did this once, then gave up. She stated the goal of treatment was "maintenance," not healing. Since my mother was declining, her wound would not heal. This was a hard pill for me to swallow. I had to let it go.

On my unit the usual pressure sores are on the coccyx (base of the spine). We would turn patients right, left, and on their back. Wounds were checked daily, usually during a bed bath or peri-care. Seeing wounds improve was inspiring. A patient's swollen body with weeping skin was distressing and indicated the body was giving up. We still do our best even if efforts were futile. Nurses in hospitals are held to a higher level of accountability to their patients than those working in long-term care.

Hygiene and wound care are visible evidence that nurses care about their patients. Knowledge alone is not enough. Dedication to the healing process is a personal commitment.

CHAPTER 7

To Break or Not to Break

Is it time for a break yet? According to our nurses' union contract, nurses are entitled to breaks. However, the legalese doesn't indicate exactly how much. Depends on who you talk to. It can be interpreted as 90 minutes or 110 minutes in total for a 12-hour shift. It's only a 20-minute discrepancy.

When I first began nursing, the breaks were scheduled as first or second break. This made no sense to me. I was never ready to have a morning break at 9:30, when I was still doing medications. Meanwhile, others lived by the clock. I resisted and ended with my first break of the day at 11:00 for an early lunch. I usually only took an hour as I had so many tasks waiting to be done. I also hoped I'd have another break in the evening.

The irony here is that no one enforces time limits on breaks. It's up to the discretion of nurses when they take breaks (and how long they are) as long as their patients are covered. Some nurses do take advantage of this, especially on night shift. Meanwhile, other nurses are so busy some days that a short break for lunch is all they feel comfortable doing.

The truth is that nurses are passive-aggressive about their powerlessness in this job. We don't get adequate pay for the responsibilities of vulnerable patients and the work we do in the hospital setting. We don't get adequate resources or support to take care of patients to our professional or our own moral standards. So, some nurses may take longer breaks.

Most nurses keep a water bottle or covered cup of water in the charting room. It's to hydrate us and keep us going when break time is far away or illusive. We need water to be able to communicate (to prevent a dry throat) with our patients. They get scheduled two cups of water and on demand water as well.

Many nurses also refuse to do daily government stats for this reason too. How does providing percentages of time allocated to each patient give meaningful data to the government? The previous government's nursing workload stats, GRASP Workload Measurement System (WMS), at least asked about actual tasks done for each patient. It is at times like this that nurses feel overregulated and overworked for no good reason. Lack of respect goes both ways.

When I was a student doing my clinical rotation on other units, there didn't seem to be this stressful decision of when to break. Even my preceptor never broke a sweat about the work. I think the nature of the unit makes a huge difference. I did my pre-grad clinical in the Head and Neck unit. Most of the patients were ambulatory but had NG tubes due to oral or throat cancer. Everything was predictable and orderly. The NG tube took away the preference of meals and timing of medications.

In hindsight, I should have applied for a nursing position there instead of Neurosurgery. I certainly would have had an easier nursing career. Breaks certainly contribute to the wellbeing of a critical thinking nurse.

CHAPTER 8

Access to Patients and Information

Pre-pandemic, visiting hours were wide open in our unit. Two visitors at any time. We were told that after the experience with Severe Acute Respiratory Syndrome (SARS) in 2003, patients and their families complained about the No Visitor Policy during that four-month outbreak. And so, the pendulum swung the other way.

Nurses need family members for medical histories, emotional support for patients, and (if able) to help with minor care like oral care or feeding. Keeping patients engaged with someone familiar helps recovery and alerts staff to changes in cognition or behaviour.

On the other hand, visitors can add stress to the nurse's obligations to other patients. They ask questions that should be reserved for the doctor. For example, what did the CT say? Or let's put the patient's own clothes on or their own pull-ups (when he/she can't move their legs). They may do that in nursing homes, but not in hospitals. Despite being proactive, visitors may take up the nurse's valuable time and energy.

Access to information can now be found on the hospital's patient portal website. It's a mixed blessing too. In signing up, there is a waiver everyone clicks informing the patient he/she may get results from tests before the doctor has had a chance to discuss, sometimes even before a nurse can check online, as well.

For patients who just want to know the results of their bloodwork (i.e., the numbers) or their next appointment, it can be great. Then there are those who do an Internet search on everything and scare themselves silly because tests and scans should only be read and understood within the context of the patient's condition and medical history. After all, each patient is unique. Most have secondary medical conditions (comorbidities).

Unfortunately, these patient portals also include many hospital nursing assessments that are not useful. The Confusion Assessment Method (CAM) is a screening tool for delirium. In my experience, it is negative 99% of the time. On our unit we assess every shift. Do patients really need full transparency? Maybe get a focus group to determine what patients and families want and need to know. The Internet already has enough information overload and misinformation as it is. Outpatients are already limited to what they can access via patient portals. Be smart and more selective.

In 1993 the Supreme Court of Canada said the hospital medical records belong to the patient, but the physical records belong to the hospital. At one time, if requested, a patient could read their paper chart if a nurse was present. (To prevent additions or deletions to this legal document). Today with online charting becoming the new standard, what physical records are left to fight over?

Patients accessing medical information seems to be on the rise. Both can add burden to the nurse's duties and responsibilities. Perhaps future hospitals will be built with beds with patients' screens for family interactions like the screens for passengers on airplanes. And maybe doctors need to be more available via video calls to answer patients' questions if they can't come to the unit. Why not dream big?

CHAPTER 9

Hospital Admissions

Perhaps we should go back to how patients are admitted to hospitals? At my hospital most patients are admitted by a doctor after being assessed in the Emergency Department (ED). Of course, all incoming patients are first seen by the ED reception desk, then assessed and prioritized by the triage nurse. The initial VS will be included in this assessment. The triage desk also gets advance notice of incoming ambulances with critical patients.

Depending on the area of medical concern, the appropriate resident of that medical service assesses the patient, orders scans, or bloodwork, and if admitted, frequency of vitals or neuro assessments, diet, and maybe an intravenous solution. Much will depend on how unstable a patient may be. He/she might be sent to ICU, a step-down unit, or a unit (like mine) for stable patients. In dire circumstances, patients may be sent straight to surgery as soon as possible. It all depends on multiple factors.

There's a big push to clear the admitted patients from the ED within 48 hours. The media reports only the wait times for patients not yet seen by doctors, not the admitted patients waiting for a bed. All units feel the pressure to get patients better and moved to the next appropriate level of care. So, a new admission to our unit can happen at any time, but usually after the morning meeting of managers (or Charge Nurses on weekends) of all the units. Only the patient's name, gender, diagnosis, and the staff doctor of the medical service who admitted the patient are given at this time.

These patients usually come on a stretcher pushed by a porter, and then are transferred to a bed. The nurse assigned to the patient assists unless the PCA is available. This is when the nurse first finds out how mobile the patient is and what safety measures are needed.

Next is the admission assessment and various tasks after an introduction to the patient. The patient's whiteboard is completed with the current date, the nurse's name, and any other timely information. Doing vital signs is the first task as it gives a baseline of what is normal for this person. (Our unit doesn't get an ED nurse's handover report.) Then the neuro assessment is done to determine any cognitive deficits or limb weaknesses.

Both types of assessments are important for monitoring changes in health status, but also for safety. For example, very low blood pressure can cause dizziness while getting out of bed and cause a fall. And the confusion of not recognizing one is in hospital or of one's diminished abilities, can also lead to trying to leave the bed independently while confused or weakened.

Then the embarrassing swab for Methicillin-resistant Staphylococcus aureus (MRSA) must be done. Not a great way to meet a new patient. However, this infection is very contagious, and staff may inadvertently spread it to other patients. The housekeeper's cleaning is therefore very important to keep these bacteria away. So is the frequent handwashing of all nurses, PCAs, therapists, and doctors. That's why hand sanitizer dispensers are found everywhere.

The MRSA test is done for all in-patients as it's a nosocomial infection (common to acquire in hospital settings) easily picked up by touching surfaces. The first swab enters the nostrils, the second one both axillae (underarms), groin and perineum (the area between the vulva or scrotum and the anus). The results will come back the following day. If they don't, the swab may have been lost or not actually done. It then must be redone.

If this test comes back positive, the patient gets a private room and is put in isolation with contact precautions. Most patients who already have MRSA may have no symptoms and be unaware they have it. However, it can affect how their wounds heal and can cause consequences for the new patient and whoever shares that room and its washroom. Most rooms in my unit are two-bedded. We have two ward rooms with four beds. Therefore, it really is an important test that is automatically ordered (computer generated) upon admission.

While doing the swab it is a good time to multi-task and do a skin assessment of immobile patients. This involves checking for scars, wounds, redness, swelling, or sites of pain. Hopefully, the patient already has a saline lock (IV access) from the ED nurse, which saves time inserting one for future IV treatments. Not all nurses have this delicate talent of threading a needle into a patent's vein (the plastic IV cannula stays, but the needle is removed), and not all patients have easily accessible veins either.

Before leaving the patient, the nurse needs to orient the patient to the call bell, the bed function buttons, personal storage, the washroom, or any other useful devices like a urinal. I also like to provide a fresh cup of water.

If the patient is mobile, then orientation includes the Patient's Kitchenette (pantry), where there's a sink, filtered water machine, microwave, and refrigerator. The fridge is a shared space for patients to save small amounts of food. Their food should be labelled with the owner's name and date. The honour system usually works. After a month, it's tossed out, or sooner, if gone bad.

The full orientation involves other areas of the unit. It includes the shared wheelchair accessible shower area, and the mini shower room dedicated for patients with epilepsy.

The Nurses' Station also has a sign-out book for patients for when they leave the unit to visit the food court downstairs. If a patient is in a wheelchair, the person pushing the wheelchair usually tells the staff where they are going. This logbook helps us to mostly locate the independent patient when needed for medications, tests, nurse, or doctor.

If the nurse still has time available, she/he will return to the patient once the written doctor's orders are reviewed, and any immediate orders carried out. The next task is the Nursing Admission Assessment, which is eight pages long. It is a mix of current and past medical history, home health, and social situation.

If the patient is alert and oriented, it can be completed in 15 minutes with no distractions or interruptions. Then it needs to be entered online at some point. Ideally this questionnaire is completed directly online via mobile computers. In my experience the WOWs were not 100% reliable when I used them.

If the patient is unconscious, confused, or there is a language barrier, the questionnaire may have to wait until a partner or family member can answer these personal questions. Therefore, the Nursing Admission Assessment may only be partially completed.

How useful are these assessments? When were they last revised? I know nurses are told they must be completed within the first 24 hours of admission. It is a checkbox on the Pre-op Checklist. Yet I have never seen a doctor read them or refer to them. If some detail is important, the nurse must verbally tell the doctor, or pass it on to the Charge Nurse to do so.

Another twist to the admission process is the *bed-spaced patient*, who has no available bed on the appropriate unit. This is a patient from ED or another unit if overflowing. They are usually a stable medicine patient with a common gastrointestinal (GI) or urological condition. However, my nurses are specialized in neurological conditions and procedures.

Pre-COVID, most of the bed-spaced patients were spinal patients. Their unit is next door, and their doctors are slightly more accessible. But these patients required spinal cord testing, which we rarely do. I know I had to use the anatomy map for the dermatomes I needed to test. So, my unit didn't like spinal patients for this reason. And the reverse was also true. Spinal nurses were afraid of neurology patients with epilepsy.

Now imagine you are designated a *hallway patient*. This is not acceptable to most Canadians, unless it is a Code Orange (mass casualty situation). It's still a bad idea, but nurses have no say.

Hallway patients are admitted patients who have waited in ED for a bed in the appropriate unit. Their time in ED is up (government incentives) and if ambulatory, are set up with a bed in front of the Nurses' Station. Privacy is provided by a screen.

It is a gamble how long this patient will be left vulnerable or uncomfortable this way. Maybe one to several hours as discharges can have unpredictable delays. Is it any wonder that some patients decide, after days in ED, this was another insult? I have seen two patients leave Against Medical Advice (AMA) because they felt it was unacceptable and that another hospital would be better. Perhaps they were right.

We all have certain expectations of what may be involved with a hospital stay. The first part is getting admitted. If we have no prior experience, then we rely on what we've seen on TV or other streaming services. I have no recent hospital experience as a patient. All I can say is the patient's experience in the Emergency Department is different from the other admitted patients' units.

CHAPTER 10

Patients with Epilepsy

On my nursing unit we also had a specialized epilepsy mini unit. These are elective admissions—patients volunteer to stay in the hospital to get diagnosed with epilepsy and to locate the origin of their seizure activity in the brain.

Epilepsy is a condition where chronic, unprovoked, transient abnormal brain activity causes a seizure. Seizures have many different manifestations. They may appear as zoning out, staring, overwhelming emotional sensations, physical shaking or sudden muscle weakness, and dropping. Some people have warning signs that something is about to happen and can get to a safe position (like sitting down). Others are not so lucky.

All seizures are not epileptic seizures. There are many causes of seizures that can be related to fever, hypoglycemia (low blood sugar), vitamin deficiency, drugs, alcohol, or heart condition. And then there are idiopathic epileptic seizures, where the cause is unknown. Therefore, it is important to determine if the patient's seizures are epileptic, by having evidence of changes of brain waves on an electroencephalogram (EEG).

Triggering a seizure in hospital can be tricky. That's part one of the hospital stay. To help this along the epilepsy doctor will reduce the patient's home antiepileptic medication until seizures begin. Most of these patients are independent and mobile. So, they may not be in their room, or on video, or their cable may accidentally be disconnected from their seizure box.

Nurses assigned to these patients need to be able to drop whatever they are doing to respond to a seizure. There is an epilepsy technician watching both the live EEG and video, who may be first to press the seizure alarm to alert the nurse. The patient can also press the seizure alarm attached to the seizure box. The nurse's priority is to make certain the patient is safe, then connected, and then visible on video.

I was originally trained to ensure the patient's face and legs were visible, because it may be characteristic of the seizure. Also, some seizures may manifest first in the face with a twitch or droop.

Other nurses were trained to automatically put the patient in rescue position (on their side), which may obscure some of the seizure appearance. If someone's lips turn blue, of course I would apply nasal prongs for oxygen. If someone has excessive saliva, then suctioning is appropriate. I still think putting a patient in rescue position before the seizure is over is premature and may miss certain seizure details.

I once had a patient's spouse interfere during a monitored seizure event. She was screaming at me to reposition him immediately. I believe she thought he'd die otherwise (as implied on TV). When I refused after assessing the patient, based on my knowledge and experience, she went ahead to do what she was trained to do in the community.

The patient was safe in bed, and I was at the bedside monitoring the situation. I believe she ruined the video, but I never found out if this was true. Another reason to have multiple recorded events.

Part two of the epilepsy hospital stay is determining the location of the seizure origin in the brain. There is a possibility for brain surgery to stop seizures from starting. However, the brain has areas of high importance (like speech, motor, and sensory) that any interference with would be detrimental to the patient. Epilepsy surgery is meant to improve the quality of life of patients.

To help locate the origin of the seizure, the patient is set up with about 30 electrodes, glued to the scalp, with long wires attached to a box (like a heart Holter monitor). When the patient is at bedside, a cable from the wall is connected to this box, and video monitoring from the ceiling is activated. Patients are advised not to sit with their back to the camera. The video is meant to confirm seizure location in the brain to the observed seizure expression.

Sometimes there isn't enough data to be accurate, and an extra step involves surgery to insert depth electrodes into the crevasses of the brain. The patient returns at some point in the future, six months maybe, and is admitted as a neurosurgery patient, but has a bed in the epilepsy unit for further monitoring.

This is more challenging for the patient as he/she has no small seizure box to disconnect. Instead, the numerous internal electrodes are attached to a heavy cable box on a pole on wheels that has a long cable (long enough to get to the washroom).

I believe nurses on my unit have the best nurse-doctor working relationship with these doctors. Neither neurology nor neurosurgery residents stay longer than two weeks and three months, respectively, since my hospital is a teaching hospital. But epilepsy doctors are a small group of staff doctors who rotate every week or so.

The epilepsy team also includes a dedicated NP who coordinates admissions, does the admitting epilepsy interview, and orders medications and the discharges. I can't forget the EEG technicians who have always helped the nurses in the past. Usually, it has been for technical and safety support, but also moral support when things don't go exactly as planned. Plus, the nurses cover the technician's break on night shift.

Since the epilepsy service has specific goals (i.e., determine if it's a seizure, then its location), protocols and medical directives have been set up long ago. This has helped nurses be autonomous in their practice and offers predictability amid the uncertainty of seizures. Patients with epilepsy should be comforted by this knowledge.

CHAPTER 11

Hospital Discharges

At the end of a hospital stay the patient is discharged. It is primarily the team's (staff doctor and resident's) decision, based on why the patient was admitted. It used to be straightforward. It still can be, but, over the years, patient and family satisfaction has increasingly influenced this final transition.

If a patient was admitted to the hospital to get their medications adjusted for PD or epilepsy, then everyone is happy to go home quickly. Home—if that's where the patient came from. We all assume that's the happy ending.

Most patients come from a variety of "home" situations. If the patient can't go home, it delays discharge and blocks a bed for a new patient. That's where our unit's social worker helps sort out the family and living issues. It's common for families to avoid planning for a nursing home or an assisted living residence for their elderly parent, or for a spouse to be unwilling to take back their more impaired partner.

On our unit we have had several patients waiting for months or years for a preferred nursing home. Previously, one had to choose three nursing homes, and the first one that offered a bed, you took. It seemed to work.

I don't recall the specifics of the major change in policy, only that it happened after my mother was already in her nursing home. A provincial politician got upset about her mother's situation of first bed offer and changed the rules. I don't remember her name except it happened after 2007 (and an Internet search was unsuccessful). Back then a patient could wait for their first pick at the hospital, even an acute care hospital like mine. Total control of choosing a nursing home and where to wait for it was given to the patient's family.

And now the Conservative provincial government is swinging the pendulum the other way, telling patients and families they have no choice at all. The new Bill 7 is called "More Beds, Better Care Act, 2022." Discharged patients will get the first nursing home bed available (I assume within Toronto and the GTA). This is temporary while they wait for their preferred location. However, some nursing homes are culture specific and may involve residents' first language, familiar foods, and religious celebrations.

I don't see how the government can then force families to pay the nursing home fees for a decision they didn't agree to. The current alternative (threat) is to charge these families $400 per day ($2,800/week) while overstaying their hospital visit. That's more than the cost of a private hospital room. It's more than the cost of the nursing home ($1800/month).

Is it any wonder that Bill 7 is being challenged? The Ontario Health Coalition and the Advocacy Centre for the Elderly have filed a Notice of Application to the Ontario Superior Court of Justice. Liam Casey's article "Ontario nursing home law violates Charter, advocates allege in lawsuit" is the follow-up to the initial media blitz of November 21, 2022 (*The Canadian Press*, April 13, 2023).

I am very grateful that my family agreed to place my mother, who had dementia, into a Ukrainian nursing home nearby while she was still living at home. My sister and separated brother were living with my parents at the time. I had persuaded this brother to move back home when I moved out. Both siblings were both busy working from home.

However, there were challenges, including getting my father to cooperate with community resources while we waited for the nursing home bed. We had my mother signed up for an adult day program, where she was picked up in the morning and returned in the afternoon. That lasted until she became too aggressive. Then we had a personal care worker come to bathe her and feed her lunch. My father didn't like strangers in the house. Although he never asked directly, I felt pressured to move back home, or at least spend more time there.

We had chosen two places and got our second choice. When our first choice became available a year later, my mother was settled, and we were satisfied with how things worked out. Still, I felt like I visited her the most despite my family living only 10 minutes away.

One of the hardest and highest-risk discharges for nurses are those where the person lives on the street and has no supportive family or friends. It's like you know you're setting up that person to fail. Ironically, the unhoused patient is eager to leave the hospital. On paper, the patient is discharged to a shelter he/she had frequented in the past. What happens afterwards is anyone's guess.

Patients are not always back at their baseline after treatment or surgery. They may be worse off, or requiring neuro or physical rehabilitation, or additional cancer treatments elsewhere. These are easier discharges as waiting for rehab beds is relatively shorter. Cancer treatments are for those whose life expectancy and/or quality of life can be improved. Most treatments in Toronto are outpatient appointments, since Princess Margaret Hospital has limited beds for immobile patients.

In an ideal world, the doctor knows when to discharge the patient after treatment. At one point, we had a standardized care pathway for patients with pituitary tumours. However, it was never used, to my knowledge. I don't think the residents knew about this preprinted doctor's order form.

Each patient had different outcomes after surgery. All the "pit. tumour" patients had at least one day after surgery in a step-down unit. But post-operative complications of diuresis (excessive urination) can occur days later, or vision deficits can continue. Adjusting steroid medication, monitoring urine output, and testing for visual fields deficits are some of the common and required aftercares.

With surgical patients, in general, it depends on the type of neurosurgery and what is indicated in the pathology report. If the patients have no deficits, they can be sent home to wait for this report. Four days after surgery, most skin incisions with staples or sutures don't need a dressing and are left open to air to heal (nursing best practice).

Often, nurses wait for the doctor's order to discharge, the Discharge Summary and prescriptions to be written. The patient may be told at the morning doctors' rounds about leaving, but the paperwork takes anywhere from 30 minutes to hours to complete. Meanwhile, the patient may have already called family to be picked up.

This is stressful for everyone. It used to be the Neurosurgery Discharge Summary was written much later and faxed to the family doctor. Now Nurse Practitioners (NPs), who work closely with the doctors in the clinic and on the units (Monday to Friday), write these summaries. After Rounds, the doctors go to the Operating Room, and the NPs to the Neurosurgery Clinic. And the unit nurse gets to calm down the patient and explain the discharge procedure and the usual delays.

The nurse also must remove any remaining saline locks on the patient; assess wounds; change dressings if within the first four days of surgery; check and retrieve any home medications or personal valuables given at admission for safekeeping; then, do a last check to make sure cell chargers or other personal items aren't left at the bedside.

Once the patient is ready to leave, it helps if the patient's family member is present for discharge instructions. It's all written down in the unit's nursing cover sheet and the Discharge Summary. However, the nurse still gives a verbal presentation of the highlights of the report and the next clinical appointment.

The nurse shouldn't have to proofread the Discharge Summary. I used to only read the last section about follow-up appointment dates. However, doctors are tired or busy, or just don't know the patient well for whom they are writing the summary. I started reviewing to make sure that they wrote the correct pronoun after such an occurrence. Nothing is worse than a doctor using "he" or "his" when the patient is female. It makes one wonder if the summary is about this patient at all.

After the nurse speaks with the patient and family member, it is also an opportunity for any clarification and other questions. Sometimes there's a last-minute request for a different kind of medication, which would involve another delay as it involves contacting the doctor or NP.

For surgical patients the nurse provides the unit's cover sheet, the Discharge Summary, staple remover if applicable, and the prescription. For the other services, the patient just gets the cover sheet, and if needed, a prescription, and waits for follow-up appointments if required.

There isn't much time between a discharge and a new patient (whether a new admission or a transfer from another unit). The nurse is also expected to strip the bed. Once the housekeeper has cleaned and sanitized the bed, tables, surfaces, and the floor is dry, then the bed is available for the next patient.

CHAPTER 12

Continuing Education

Continuing education is required for all nurses. In hospitals nurses must get recertified annually for CPR or any higher cardiac/emergency training required for their unit. The CPR courses are hands-on and offered after work hours. Usually, one must find a class on one's own at an organization like The Michener Institute, or someone can organize one at the hospital for a group of nurses or colleagues. I did this for many years.

In addition, the hospital has many eLearning courses that nurses must complete annually, and some require passing the accompanying quizzes. However, these courses require dedicated time and quiet space. That can't happen in a noisy and busy unit, with interruptions at any time, ringing call bells, or passersby.

Bedside nurses are paid by the hour, but this doesn't reflect the education we have to maintain on our own personal time. It would be one thing if we were paid by a salary, which one would assume included professional development.

The clinical educator for our unit works regular office hours Monday to Friday. She is available for questions and/or supervising bedside procedures that nurses do infrequently or have never done before.

There is so much to know about chest tubes, lumbar puncture drains, changing dressings for central lines, or inserting a saline lock to access a Port-a-Cath, for instance. Some patients with cancer come from home with this port embedded in their skin. Nurses need to access them for IV medication and bloodwork. It feels like the skills list is never-ending.

I remember a doctor ordering a new medication on our unit, Octaplex®, on a Saturday. It reverses the effects of anticoagulants (blood thinners) like Warfarin. The patient needed to go to surgery as soon as possible. This medication is often used in ED, but the patient got admitted to our floor quickly instead. The pharmacy department sent up the medication in the packaging with the instructions inside. I was so nervous that I could barely read and understand what was in my hands. Consulting my colleagues, I found the appropriate YouTube video (from the manufacturer). Seeing it done gave me the confidence to follow through and administer it.

As you may have guessed, I relied heavily on the clinical educator and our unit pharmacist throughout the years. There are times when you must get the medication or procedure done quickly and correctly the first time.

There's a lot of talk about *critical thinking* skills in nursing school. But I don't believe critical thinking can be taught in a textbook. It requires exposure to multiple situations and stressful on-the-spot decision making. Practice only makes better decisions, not perfect ones.

In my eLearning inbox, I came across something like a "Non-Disclosure Agreement" (NDA) in 2016 and 2018. The course was called Annual Privacy, which I didn't see in other years. I should have asked someone about this at the time. However, I think it was a mandatory course and I'm the type of person who likes to clear my inbox. I started reading the first one, which covered patient confidentiality. Why did I have to sign this if it's already part of my requirement as a registered nurse with the College of Nurses?

I signed it not once, but twice. I never got a copy, I never tried to print it, and I never saw the word "NDA" on it. I asked Human Resources in 2022 and was told it wasn't in my personnel file. In addition to this, during the

COVID-19 forum talks, the hospital was upset staff were discussing corporate affairs publicly online. I also heard nurses complained about ONA negotiations on Facebook. I was too busy working my essential job to even think about doing this.

CHAPTER 13

Awkward Personal Questions

Often patients would ask their nurse personal questions. I guess they thought since we know a lot about them, these questions would balance out the knowledge the nurse had of them. However, my knowledge as their nurse is mostly about their medical condition. When I put on my nurse's uniform, I am their nurse, a professional, not a private citizen who can perhaps easily navigate personal questions by leaving or refusing to answer. This social etiquette works well in regular conversations outside of the hospital setting. However, it could be I'm just naturally more sensitive or private.

I have always had a hard time answering these questions. The patients always asked, "Are you married, do you have children?" As soon as I said, "No," the follow-up question was "Why not?" Isn't that rude? As if I knew the real answer or was assertive enough to avoid answering. This is the opposite of the TMI (too much information) behaviour often shared online by celebrities and wannabes. I find it invasive.

The most frequent question, however, was, "Where are you from?" I guess my name didn't sound Canadian enough even though I knew three other women named Zenia. (And not zinnia like the flower, or Xena: Warrior Princess—the TV series). I would answer, "I'm from Toronto" or "I was born in Toronto." Then they would backtrack and try again with, "What's your family background?"

I had to pause for reflection and decide how much to disclose. Walking away makes me uncomfortable unless I have a real excuse. If the patient had a European background, I might answer directly. However, if a patient spoke Russian or had a Russian sounding name, then I needed to proceed carefully to avoid creating possible obstacles to the nurse-patient relationship.

As a child I was taught Russia was the enemy of Ukraine. At the time, Ukraine was still part of the Soviet Union (USSR), but the second-largest republic. Ukraine was known as the breadbasket of Europe for its wheat and fertile black soil. The country was briefly independent in 1918, before it was absorbed into the Soviet Union. So, my father was elated when Ukraine became independent again in 1991 after the disintegration of the USSR.

Many historical events like Holodomor (the Great man-made Famine of 1932–33), and the explosion of the Chernobyl nuclear power plant in 1986 showed Russia didn't regard Ukraine as a cherished Soviet republic, or a friendly neighbouring country. The current Russian invasion of Ukraine (2022–) is another example. Nonetheless, as a nurse, I kept my personal opinions and biases locked down. As an adult, I have tried to treat each person as an individual.

Then there was one patient who was collecting accents. On our unit we had nurses with diverse backgrounds. He asked all the staff to stop by so he could guess and identify these accents. Maybe he had a notebook like a birder. When I got there, he sent me away. I had no accent, so I must be Canadian. I had mixed feelings about that.

When I was a child, my best friend said she was more Canadian than me. One time she even said, suddenly out of the blue, I had an accent. She was being mean. However, she continued this verbal attack. Her main argument wasn't based on her being one month older than me, but that her family came from Newfoundland.

At the time, I thought she was right, and I felt inferior to her for a while. I wanted to be more Canadian or British like her. My parents had only come to Canada in 1948. However, years later I realized that Newfoundland and Labrador weren't even part of Canada until 1949. Therefore, I was more Canadian than her. I thought I won this one-upmanship.

Unfortunately, decades later, as I went through my parents' documents, I discovered they didn't get their Canadian citizenship until 1962. I don't think being landed immigrants counts. So, my friend was right after all.

However, in retrospect, is this even a legitimate statement or question? An adult certainly would never pose this question but might infer it like my patients did. Was collecting accents just a harmless hobby for that patient? Maybe, this question should instead be reserved for food, not people. For example, is maple syrup more Canadian than peameal bacon (round bacon with a cornmeal edge)? I vote yes.

In my work as a nurse everyone is Canadian or from Ontario (for hospital insurance purposes), unless told otherwise. Accents don't automatically reveal citizenship. I'm sure collecting accents was meant to be inoffensive and my unit had many of them floating about. The diverse background of staff doesn't devalue the nursing work being done. We were all there for the same purpose. Being Canadian is a source of pride and sensitivity for me when the wrong question is asked. The nurse's focus should remain on the patient, and not be reciprocated.

CHAPTER 14

Safety for Everyone

Safety is a major concern in every work environment, especially in hospitals. There are eLearning courses on how to properly move or transfer patients. Common sense dictates how to prevent slips on wet floors. However, the human factor of the patient, the staff, or anyone else is totally unpredictable at times. Just think of someone with a dripping coffee walking in the hallway totally unaware. It happens more often than you think.

In my experience, most patient falls occur while trying to get out of bed to go to the washroom. Spills of water from the patient's cup (despite having a lid) on the floor happen a lot. The nurse is usually first on site to dry the area with towels or bed sheets, and then to call housekeeping to finish up mopping missed spots. The housekeeper then ends with putting up a "wet floor" sign. But the nurse begins with securing the area, checking the patient(s), then making it safer for everyone.

While getting up, the patient may become incontinent and slip in his/her own urine. Or he/she can have a seizure enroute to the washroom, hitting his/her head on the floor, or in the washroom, or the shower room. A fall can happen anywhere and for any reason.

Nurses are also victims of injuries. If the nurse is rushing to get to the patient, there can be unseen obstacles on the floor, behind a privacy curtain between beds, or the same wet spill. From the minor injuries of bruises and muscle or tendon strains, to back spasms or being hit by a patient who is pos-tictal, confused, or just angry and uncooperative, nurses are a moving target.

Needlestick injuries are rare but have potentially serious consequences. These occur if the needle was used on a patient first, then the nurse or other staff get pricked afterwards by accident. Ideally, the used needle is disposed of immediately in the yellow Sharps container. However, anything can happen.

We didn't always have retractable needles. Patients can move or jerk during the injection. A needle thrown into the Sharps may bounce back at the user's hand. Someone may have thoughtlessly put the used needle into the garbage. Sometimes the retractable needle doesn't fully retract. You know this first by feeling a prick on your finger, then seeing the blood.

The protocol for a needle stick injury requires notifying the appropriate supervisor or Charge Nurse to get the patient's doctor to speak with the patient to consent to immediate bloodwork. This is to test for HIV and hepatitis B (HBV). Meanwhile, the injured party should squeeze the pricked area to allow any contaminated blood out, run cold water over it, then cover it with a BAND-AID® and go back to work.

Lifting patients, on the other hand, is a repetitive action for nurses and can cause problems like chronic tendonitis. Unless there is acute pain, one usually doesn't report it.

In fact, while working, most nurses don't feel their bodies because they are super focused on attending to their patients. For this reason, most wash-room breaks for nurses happen at the beginning or the end of the shift and during meal breaks.

This reminds me of a cartoon of a nurse on roller skates, with a stetho-scope around her neck, and a urinary bag hanging from her scrub pants' pocket. The cartoonist got that right.

As the COVID-19 era emerged the situation for hospital nurses became more problematic. Nurses had to wear personal protective equipment to prevent catching or spreading the respiratory virus. Wearing a procedure face mask or the N95 mask also reduced the opportunities for drinking water. The face shield or goggles got steamed up if one wore glasses too. It became harder for patients to hear the nurse speak due to the layers of protection. So the nurse would speak louder or come closer to the patient to be heard.

Therefore, although the protection nurses wore was for the safety of everyone, it also made the work of nurses more burdensome and awkward.

CHAPTER 15

Self-Care and Energy Cleansing

Time for oneself was never a priority or even on my list of tasks. Self-care for nurses happened at home. That's when we had a safe space to try to forget the stresses of the hospital workday. It wasn't always successful for me.

A long drive home with the music blaring was one of my therapies. Eating my missed meals was emotional eating rather than good therapy. Decompressing was sometimes impossible if exhausted. Worse was being so tired one couldn't sleep. Flipping between day shift and night shift didn't help. How I hated night shift, but someone had to do it, preferably not me.

My sister Maria moved in with me during the first year of the pandemic. I had an empty spare bedroom. It seemed an ideal solution for my brothers, but I never considered what the consequences could be for me. I thought I was helping her out, but her presence drove me insane. I felt trapped by her numerous boxes of possessions. It literally made me itch having her in my space.

I developed a rash on the right side of my neck and thought I had shingles. The doctor I saw disagreed with me but gave me a cream. He also gave in to my request for the shingles vaccine. It was months before my sister finally moved out. I sighed with extreme relief, but felt guilty I couldn't tolerate her presence. I don't know where she moved as she stopped talking to me, and my brothers didn't share her new location. We had never been close as sisters, but this was a new low.

I always used massage, which was a group benefit. However, when I first started nursing, I needed a doctor's note to endorse needing a massage for the insurance company to approve the benefit. Do they not know what hospital nurses do? Eventually the nurses' union got rid of this requirement. But the annual limit of $400 remained the same. I was always maxed out by May. Once in a blue moon we also had free chair massages for 10 minutes on the unit. I don't think I would've lasted long in nursing without massages.

When the body totally relaxes, a peaceful mind follows. That's what I learned in meditation and yoga so many years ago. However, if verbally abused, it can mess up one's mental, emotional, spiritual, and physical aspects.

Unfortunately, some patients or family members yell or demand things from nurses. I remember one spouse demanded bed sheets be changed daily because her husband sweats. I asked if that was done at home. She claimed she did, but I was skeptical. My personal nursing practice was to change bed sheets for visible stains or wetness. Why do you think beds have bed pads placed where incontinence occurs?

Some nurses bully other nurses and managers seem indifferent or just expect the nurses to work it out between themselves. Words can hurt, but the scars aren't visible. Verbal abuse accumulates and demeans one's self-worth and the confidence to do the job. Ironically, during the COVID-19 crisis the additional layers of masks and face shields, plus limited sitting in the staff lounge, deterred verbal abuse.

There's a lot of talk about mental health these days. Support is available everywhere, but as a nurse I needed immediate support, instead of making a telephone appointment (previous bad experience). I thought we had a hotline. Some employers have outsourced this employee benefit. I don't like the idea of talking to a stranger, let alone talking about it much later. It feels like regurgitation and is embarrassing too. I don't know any nurse who does any kind of therapy as it's a very personal and private process. I guess I'm still impatient about some things.

When I was much younger, I went to see a therapist. He agreed I was stressed at home but did not recommend anything or suggest a follow-up. I literally paid him to let me vent. I guess I was just a hormonal teenager to him. I was very dissatisfied with this experience. Instead, the next time I was stressed, I went for a long run until I rid myself of my strong emotions. I felt much better too. I also started writing in a journal whenever I was angry, overwhelmed, or sad.

Luckily, my nursing colleagues let me vent frequently about work (and for free). This was in my last years when I felt I was in a comfortable space with my coworkers. We were all in the same boat. Others gave their opinions and vented to a lesser degree, so I waited for my turn when I could during staff meetings. Some nurses were naturally outspoken and spoke with confidence. I, on the other hand, spoke from frustration and powerlessness. It was a coping mechanism.

At other times the hospital's Spiritual Care professionals gave me unexpected solace and understanding. Usually, I called them for patients or their families, but they would touch base with me too. I am grateful to have been supported by all these uplifting individuals.

I also believe energy builds up in hospital rooms as it does in individuals. I have experienced this with my Reiki and Therapeutic Touch background. My regret is that Spiritual Care wouldn't clear the accumulated negative energies in the patients' rooms. I was told they weren't allowed to bless (or cleanse) a unit as someone might get offended. Some rooms had more deaths or stranger energy than others. (And, no I have never seen or felt a ghost in the rooms of the departed.) I snuck in my Tibetan bells a few times when the rooms were empty. I had no time for Reiki for my patients, but a healing energy environment should somehow have been possible.

I would have preferred my whole unit to have been blessed or spiritually cleansed by Spiritual Care. Any religion or practice would have been welcome. It would have been even better than duct cleaning. Both nurses and patients benefit when nurses are cared for as well.

CHAPTER 16

Death of a Patient

Unexpected deaths are the worst. I have heard of older generations believing anyone admitted to a hospital was expected to die. It's not true because of newer technology, medication or treatments, Code Blue protocols, CPR training, or closer observations by nurses. However, nurses can't be everywhere. Sometimes it may just be your time.

One time, while talking to a patient, I had taken a few steps and turned around to get my VS machine, then discovered she had died. She had Alzheimer's disease and her family had previously agreed to a code status of "No CPR" (previously known as "DNR"—do-not-resuscitate order). A nearby doctor heard me and started CPR on her, despite my telling him her code status. Once someone else confirmed it, he just stopped. I didn't know you could do that, I mean, stop once you started compressions.

I also couldn't understand how I was more upset than her daughter about the patient dying. She gave *me* comfort, with a hug and by confirming it was okay. She knew her mother was dying slowly already and had made peace with it. It was only much later with my own mother, who also had Alzheimer's, that I understood the long goodbye families face with such diseases. In my own mother's situation, it was a relief with deep sadness, not grief. Not the deep sorrow caused by death and the pain of loss.

Sometimes the expected deaths are easier to endure. These patients might have plans in place by the palliative team after consultation with the family. These can include reducing regular medications and giving only the necessary ones for respiratory secretions, analgesics, or antiepileptics.

Quality of death should always be considered. Watching a patient with shortness of breath is difficult, even with supplemental oxygen, but it may be part of their dying process. However, letting anyone suffer with pain is just cruel.

Yet, it's difficult not to empathize with the family who second guess what their loved one would've wanted. Some families say, "Do everything possible," even when it's obvious the body is rejecting this extra help. Giving IV fluids or enteral feeds to a body that isn't absorbing is the opposite of caring, to my mind and heart. As nurses, we are subjected to all kinds of deaths, where we play an active role.

The latest innovation of the death process in the hospitals is called Medical Assistance in Dying (MAID). This is where a competent person with an incurable disease expected to get much worse can decide to die with dignity in a medical setting. It's a quality-of-life issue versus dying quickly on one's own terms (i.e., quality of death).

Currently, it is not for patients with depression, or other mental or cognitive diseases. Although the original strict guidelines (2016) have been revised (2021) after much feedback and review. In 2023 MAID was revised again to include certain types of mental illness (like depression or personality disorders). However, the eligibility date has been delayed to March 2024 once "recommendations on protocols, guidance, and safeguards" for this complex category of sufferers are reviewed and determined to be prudent.

I saw a MAID storyline on *Transplant*, a TV medical drama (Season 3, Episode 13). The writers implied this procedure could be done within hours or days of the patient's request. No, it takes months to become eligible and to plan. It takes a team, and not a single doctor.

MAID is a controversial procedure requiring several IV medications injected via a saline lock within minutes. It is very carefully done. The patient decides which family or friends are invited to be present. Members of the MAID team, plus the unit nurse, are also there. The nurse treats the patient as a regular patient until it's time. The team bears witness as the doctor administers the medications. A debriefing happens afterwards to touch base with the team. It is a highly personal and emotional (or even spiritual) event that can affect you in unexpected ways afterwards. No staff is forced to participate, as it is all voluntary.

In Ontario, if a patient is expected to die, a nurse can pronounce death. However, this has no legal weight. Pronouncing death is not certifying death. Doctors, RNs (extended class), and NPs can certify death. In my hospital a doctor must still view the patient, and fill out the death certificate and any other forms. How soon this happens varies. The time of death is an estimate or when the doctor arrives. The doctor makes the notification to the next of kin and may ask if an autopsy is wanted. An autopsy may delay the body leaving the unit.

Either the doctor or nurse must call the Trillium Gift of Life Network to alert the organ donation organization. Anyone aged 85 or older is no longer eligible to donate. Anyone who has an infection will be declined for organs, with the exception of corneas. This notification is also documented.

If the family members are already present, the nurse waits for them to leave. Should no one be there, the doctor will have, hopefully, enquired during the call if someone was coming. Once no other family member is expected, then the patient's nurse and an assistant (another nurse or PCA) can go ahead and wash the dead patient. Any hospital devices are removed. The body is placed in a body bag and all personal valuables (if any) are put in a separate bag. The manager ensures the body is properly prepared and ID labels are where they belong (no toe tags). A porter is called—the body is transferred to a stretcher, and the porter and a security guard escort it to the hospital morgue.

Nursing is holistic. It can encompass the physical, mental, emotional, and spiritual, especially in the process of a dying patient.

PART II

WORKING AS A NURSE IN TIIE SARS/COVID ERA

CHAPTER 17

SARS and Nurse Casualties

The SARS outbreak changed my hospital temporarily in 2003. No visitors were allowed. In contrast, pre-SARS public hospitals were open to the public. No one manned the entrances. My hospital had six entrances, including the elevator from the underground parking. Some doors didn't open until 6:00 a.m. and closed at 10:00 p.m. Staff had badges with security microchips to let them in at any time.

I thought living nearby would be environmentally friendly, and "convenient." So, after SARS I moved closer to work. The hospital was 10 minutes away by car or taxi. I had no parking spot at my condominium building. Taking the streetcar would take 20 to 40 minutes, depending on if I caught one. There was no transit shelter to speak of, so I froze or got chilled from the wind off the lake. Walking was 20 minutes uphill (and sweaty).

After six years of TTC (public transit) I had to move out of the city (because Toronto housing was expensive) and began commuting by car. I would finally enjoy being warm getting to work.

I would also come early to beat the traffic; get a good parking spot; grab a coffee; go to my locker to stow my jacket and purse and collect my supplies (pens, pencils, highlighter, and eraser); walk upstairs to my unit to see my assignment; and retrieve my stethoscope from my cubbyhole. I would see some of the night staff and greet them, getting a sense of how their shift went.

In March 2020 COVID-19 changed my hospital again, but this time it became a fortress. The Emergency Department was inaccessible from inside of the hospital except for the staff with security badges. The other entrances had screeners asking the COVID-19 health screening questions and checking our staff ID. We had to wear a hospital-provided face mask once inside. And of course, wash our hands with antiseptic handwash before taking a new blue face mask.

Managers had meetings with staff prior to this escalation of security and vigilance. We were told not to wear our uniforms (or work shoes) to or from work, but to change at work. The nurses and PCAs were to change their face masks to the 3-ply medical face masks upon arrival to the unit, and to use either a face shield, goggles, or the hybrid shield/mask. We were not to use N95 masks unless our patient had COVID-19.

This was so different from how we prepared for SARS (2003). Back then, every patient was treated as if they had SARS, so staff wore N95 masks with every patient. I'm told we wore goggles, but I don't have a distinct memory of that. It would have been the protocol for airborne precautions: N95 masks, goggles, yellow isolation gowns, and gloves.

In front of each patient's room, we had somewhere to hang our isolation gown for that room and that was reused for that shift. It was also obvious when gowns were running low as we'd get disposable ones for a while. We were already handwashing prior to each patient. Hand sanitizer dispensers were everywhere. There was no change to glove use. We always had gloves in stock.

I do remember wearing the N95 mask only in the patient's room, not outside of it. And I still complained to my colleagues how I "couldn't breathe." However, no one got SARS on our unit. I'm sure it also helped that we had a No Visitor policy at the time. I really appreciated that.

Near the end of SARS, we had only one hospital entrance with a tent attached. It was set up for staff to have their temperature taken. I have a clear memory of ear thermometers being used. We still used our original oral thermometers for patients.

I also recall visiting my mother at her nursing home during the H1N1 flu season of 2009. The nurse manager tried to suggest I shouldn't visit despite no changes to their visitors' policy. She asked questions about how things were done at my hospital. I guess she was screening me. Years later she would brag in the news about how she kept her long-term care (LTC) facility COVID-free in 2020. I don't know if that's still the case in 2022 as vaccinating her staff had become an issue.

In hindsight, the SARS experience had many similarities to COVID-19. While I was doing my nursing degree, I met an ICU nurse who had contracted SARS. She said she was very lucky to have survived. However, now she had to be extra careful whenever she caught any cold or respiratory condition. I suspect she also had bouts of fatigue. I think she had post-SARS syndrome or "Long SARS" (like the current Long COVID).

As we know, many health care workers died of SARS globally. The average infection rate of HCWs was 21%. In Canada it was 43%, second highest to Vietnam at 57% as reported by Jian Xiao et al in the *Journal of Infection and Public Health*, 2020.

Toronto was one of the hotspots. Nelia Laroza, RN of North York General Hospital, died on June 29, 2003, after contracting it from a patient. She was one of the 44 health care workers (HCWs) who died of SARS in Canada.

Another nurse, Tecla Lin (Tecla-Lai Yin Lin), died July 19, 2003. She worked part-time at West Park Hospital and Toronto Rehab Institute. She had volunteered to work at the SARS unit, where infected staff from Toronto Grace Hospital were treated.

The media had always listed two nurses and a doctor as the only HCWs who died from SARS. The doctor wasn't as well-known as these two nurses. Dr. Nestor Yanga died August 13, 2003, after contact with a patient in his Scarborough clinic, the Lapsley Family Clinic. The walk-in patient had been potentially misdiagnosed at a hospital and was looking for a second opinion. The patient thought he had SARS. It turns out he was right.

Those were the only health care workers' deaths mentioned by the Canadian media. However, they missed one. Perhaps, since she died overseas, she didn't fit the category of dying from SARS in Canada. *The Toronto Star* revealed this oversight September 27, 2003, in their *SARS: Special Report—Lives We Lost.*

Adela Catalan was a nurse's aide at two retirement homes (LTC). That qualifies as a HCW. A nurse's aide is the same as a personal support worker (PSW) or PCA. She contracted SARS while caring for her roommate's mother. Unknowingly, she left for a wedding in the Philippines, where she died April 14, 2003.

I think Statistics Canada (StatCan) or the Public Health Agency of Canada (PHAC) should revise their information. It matters to call her a HCW to other PSWs or PCAs, the Filipino community, but especially to her family. There were four Canadian health care workers who died of SARS.

SARS wasn't a pandemic. It was called a viral outbreak (not an epidemic) that spread from the province of Guangdong, China to dozens of countries, including Canada. We were number 4 on this list, but our Toronto SARS outbreak (with two clusters) only lasted four months in total.

SARS started in China in November 2002. The last documented case was in April 2004 post-outbreak, in China, by a cluster of infected lab researchers (ironically researching SARS). Otherwise, the last recognized global case was in the US on July 13, 2003.

Most of the SARS cases were travel related or by close contact. Contact tracing was pretty good, or so I thought, at the time. Although fewer people got SARS than COVID-19 (8422 vs. COVID's millions), it was faster and deadlier (916 dead). There were no tests, vaccines, or cures. We had personal protection equipment (PPE) like N95 masks, quarantines, and travel restrictions.

So, if we did such a good job with SARS, why were we doing things differently this time with COVID-19?

CHAPTER 18

N95 Masks

"Lessons learned from SARS" is a phrase I kept hearing when my hospital's infection control measures for COVID-19 were being discussed. But no one explained what that meant. I really had to dig deep to find a possible answer. Most of it had to do with political hesitancy to close international travel, lack of communication between levels of government or public health, and depleting supplies of personal protective equipment (PPE). I had no idea we were running low on N95 masks (respirators) during SARS. In those days we only had one type, the white "dust masks" with the yellow elastic bands.

After SARS we started getting N95 face mask fittings to ensure efficacy. Not all faces, chins or noses are alike, therefore neither are the N95 masks you wear if you want 95% coverage. Over the years I've had different masks, and now I'm back to the "original" style 3M™ 8210 mask. So, I'm very skeptical of the public wearing any N95 mask without being properly fitted. I'm not even sure if N95 mask fitting is available to the public. The mask-fitting test involves having a chemical sprayed on your mask while under a dome and is an uncomfortable procedure.

The World Health Organization (WHO) had determined that both SARS and COVID-19 were not airborne pathogens (March 2020). Both were droplet and contact viruses only. However, in July 2020 almost 300 scientists wrote an open letter to the WHO encouraging them to update the COVID-19 guidelines to include airborne precautions based on their data. In response, the international agency agreed that *aerosolized* respiratory droplets could increase the transmission of this virus. That meant when HCWs like nurses or respiratory therapists (RTs) suctioned a patient, with or without a tracheostomy tube, they were at higher risk. Suctioning is a common procedure on my unit.

Prior to our current general acceptance of droplet and contact precautions (and sometimes airborne), the original response in January 2020 by Public Health Ontario was to include airborne isolation precautions. I remember using all three isolation signs for a short period for suspected COVID-19 patients' rooms.

By March 2020 we were down to just droplet and contact precautions, then told to put up an airborne sign and close the bedside curtains while suctioning a patient with a tracheostomy tube and for 30 minutes afterwards. It was very confusing to remember when the curtains were safe to open again. We did keep a log of suctioning details for patients with tracheostomies, but it wasn't always updated or in an obvious location (in the chart or on a wall near the bed).

During the beginning of the COVID-19 era we were told the surgical or procedural face mask was enough with goggles or a face shield. And a rumour began that there weren't enough N95 masks. Why else would managers keep the supplies of those N95 masks in their offices? I think that's why the airborne versus droplet debate really took flight for me.

I did notice some doctors wearing both the N95 mask and a medical mask over it. I also saw this combination on American ER documentaries like *Emergency: NYC* (Netflix, April 2023). I think it was to appear like everyone else with the blue mask on top. But I could see the other white mask on the edges. Maybe this was to prevent comments.

Airborne diseases like pulmonary tuberculosis (TB) are taken very seriously in the hospital setting. We always use airborne precautions for them and have special negative pressure rooms (also known as airborne infection isolation rooms) with an ante room for changing into our PPE. Almost every unit has one of these private rooms.

However, the rationale for COVID-19 not being airborne is that if the infected patient coughed, then it would infect everyone in that room. Since that wasn't supported by the research, it cannot be airborne. Perhaps, instead, it's that we don't have enough negative pressure rooms (or private rooms) and no one wants to create panic.

They also talked about the size of the COVID-19 droplet, meaning the bigger the droplet, the less likely it will travel far. COVID-19 droplets are smaller than TB droplets (virus particles are smaller than bacteria). So, that should mean COVID-19 can travel further and circulate longer in the air as if airborne, based on the droplet size theory.

I will play devil's advocate and suggest that TB would not contaminate everyone in a room. Just like COVID-19 wouldn't. I think there are many variables we are still not fully aware of at play. My mother was exposed to TB after World War II in the displaced persons' camps. She never had active TB to my knowledge, but she did get coughs and colds. Why was she only exposed to TB, but not infected?

A reasonable person (or a public relations' spin) may suggest that there is a grey area between airborne and droplet, and subsequently the *aerosolized droplets* theory came into being. The hospital curtains between patients were meant for privacy, not to prevent droplets from travelling patient to patient. How often did nurses have to secure curtains closed with either tape or a safety pin? Is this how unit outbreaks occur? Or is it the shared washroom?

In July 2020 scientists wrote an open letter to the WHO stating that COVID-19 was airborne based on the mounting scientific evidence. Over 200 experts backed this claim (*CBC News, New York Times*). Then, in December 2021, the WHO quietly agreed, as described by *Nature* on April 7, 2022. As well, the Advisory Board weighed in on April 8, 2022 in with, "The coronavirus is airborne. Why did WHO take 2 years to say so?" Their careful policy process or politics? And now, try finding clear confirmation that *COVID-19 is airborne* on the WHO's website, or any website for that matter.

Brave doctors like Dr. Nili Kaplan-Myrth stated categorically on television (September 2022) that COVID-19 is airborne. She wears her N95 mask all day long in her family practice. She's not afraid to contradict the current official medical consensus.

I'm going to be brave too. COVID-19 may be spread primarily by droplet transmission, but it is also airborne, and thirdly, transmitted by contact. Everyone has conceded to aerosols carrying the virus; however, they made it sound like a separate category from airborne transmission. I was lulled into this interpretation too. It allowed hospitals to promote medical face masks instead of N95 masks for HCWs.

We should have used the N95 masks at least until the hospital staff was vaccinated. I have a feeling that either the research wasn't supporting this yet or there was political resistance and/or interference. After all, the provincial government controlled the supply of N95 masks to the hospitals.

One cannot talk about ventilation or filtration being important without COVID-19 being airborne. If COVID-19 droplets are transmitted only by droplets, then they are too heavy and short-ranged to be helped by improved air flow. Yet there was a brief flurry of activity in hospitals and schools to enhance the quality of indoor air. Good air quality is always the healthier choice.

It's interesting that my hospital got air duct cleaning done after improved ventilation was recommended to prevent and/or reduce COVID-19 transmission. The thinking at the time was that enhanced ventilation would sweep out the COVID-19 virus droplets from contaminating surfaces, and because the virus is only airborne under specific circumstances.

I still remember Sick Building Syndrome (SBS) and Legionnaires' disease from decades before. Air quality in buildings was important for a while back then too. It fizzled because improving air quality requires investment in the infrastructure of buildings. My hospital's windows are screwed shut so I was just glad the ducts were finally cleaned on the inside.

Cleaning the air alone is not enough. After calls from staff for transparency of the availability of PPE supplies (especially N95 masks), the hospital executives did post online (for staff) which supplies were low. Kudos to them for realizing the staff's right to know, and to reduce risk and anxiety.

However, it took the Ontario Nurses' Association (ONA), and the SARS Commission's *precautionary principle* to obtain the right for staff to use the N95 mask, **whenever** they felt the patient may be infected, rather than when confirmed to be COVID-19 positive. The Ontario Chief Medical Officer of Health's *Directive #5*, which finally came out in December 2021, allows the expanded use of N95 mask to suspected, probable, or confirmed COVID-19 patients. It also reaffirmed that regulated health professionals (like nurses) were to do a point-of-care risk assessment (PCRA) with all patients and tasks. Finally, some common sense prevailed.

CHAPTER 19

Cleaning Surfaces and Hands

Everyone acknowledges that housekeeping is a vital part of maintaining cleanliness and reducing microorganisms on hospital surfaces. One of the new tasks due to COVID-19 was using bleach to clean counters, tables, and even elevator doors. Everyone needed to be brought up to speed on what surfaces bleach was contraindicated for safe use. Devices like computers, IV pumps, and VS machines require non-corrosive products for the keypads and screens.

The bleach required to be left on wet, and to dry for three minutes. How does one measure the amount to use? Of course, I've ruined several scrub pants by leaning against these counters. I refused to throw away my stained work clothes as even then I didn't know how long this new practice would be in place. Also, unlike wet floors, there were no signs for wet counters.

Some of the elevator surfaces and bathroom doors had large swaths of dried bleach marks on the stainless steel. I often wondered if this was deliberate (to show it was done), or if as with my refrigerator, it's the wrong product for the surface.

At the beginning of COVID-19, the public was very concerned about cleaning their packaged food. In fact, I don't think anyone does this anymore. As a nurse I was already in the habit of frequently washing my hands, so I never bought into the idea of buying antibacterial wipes, or washing down the plastic bag that covered my romaine lettuce. I considered that extreme behaviour.

I remember one housekeeper who was always very diligent with cleaning our unit. This was before the pandemic. It's like he had the fear of God pushing him to do his very best not to miss a spot. When it came time to get vaccinated, he declined. When it became mandatory, he declined again and lost his job. He chose to leave. I don't understand this decision, nor did he ever explain. This was a sad day for all of us. I guess he was more afraid of the COVID-19 vaccine than the virus.

The hospital supply of vaccines was prioritized to selected groups. The vaccine was offered to ICU and housekeeping staff first (not sure about ED). There was limited stock of the first available batches of the Pfizer COVID-19 vaccine. I was jealous at the time as I was not eligible. I was told later that housekeepers were prioritized because they could be asked to cover any unit in the hospital, especially evenings or weekends. And so, they were a priority. I did say they were vital to our hospital, didn't I?

Handwashing is basic hygiene, a ritual, and still people take it for granted and not wash often enough. It is one of the cardinal rules for the prevention of the spread of diseases like viruses and bacteria. Yet it's only by chance that more people don't get infected from contact transmission.

I think most people know how to wash their hands if they are visibly dirty. Yet they don't consider the invisible germs that live everywhere unless you own ultraviolet light or use bleach often. A good habit is to wash your hands before eating or after using the toilet.

When I visited my cousin in Manchester, UK, I would wash my hands before meals. She commented to her husband when I missed an opportunity or two. I'm sure she didn't mean for me to overhear. She thought I was perhaps full of myself by not walking my talk. (You're a nurse, yeah, yeah.) I never asked her to do the same, but I bet you she's washing her hands more often now since COVID-19 arrived.

Is there a right way to wash your hands? Oprah (and the CDC) would have you believe 20 seconds will make you a champion handwasher. Sing "Happy Birthday" twice for the count. Longer handwashing assumes you'll do a better job of washing. I think it just means you'll use more water and let the running water do the work. You need friction and to touch all parts of the hand and wrist.

Meanwhile, according to the WHO videos, hand hygiene is washing with soap and water, and should be 40–60 seconds, and if with alcohol sanitizer, then 20–30 seconds. This is news to me. I will try to do better.

When I was studying for my nursing diploma, we did a lot of practical units. We were taught to wash our hands with soap and water up to our elbows, the backs of our hands, between our fingers, and the tips of our fingers. Unless you're an operating room nurse or doctor, you can skip the elbows, but not the scrubbing. It isn't about the length of time spent (OR protocols are different), but the mechanical friction and the areas cleaned.

In nursing school, we had to keep our nails short and bare of nail polish. I don't know why some nurses I worked with had long painted nails or nail extensions. This is not hygienic and could break through gloves. But, unlike school, there was no reinforcement of proper nail appearance at work.

Hands are an important tool for the nurse. They need to be always kept functional, clean, and ready for action. Therefore, the options are soap and water or sanitizer.

In the hospital setting staff can't run to a sink to wash their hands all the time. There is a communal sink in the medication room, plus the one in the staff's washroom. I always hesitated to use the one in the patient's room as it's meant for the patient or on behalf of the patient's care.

The hand sanitizers outside the patients' rooms are meant for staff when hands are not visibly dirty. There is a hand sanitizing protocol for when to wash your hands before entering a patient's room, during, and after. We've even had handwashing audits by surreptitious personnel in the hallway. Each unit gets rated a percentage of compliance and compared to other units.

Audits were done monthly or less often, but these added to nurses' stress. As if my nursing job wasn't hard enough, if I had to carry something into the patient's room, I had to make a big production of washing my hands inside the room so the auditor could see. Otherwise, I would be "caught" for not following protocol. Doctors were notorious for not following protocol. And what about visitors' hands?

I have yet to see anyone wash their hands with sanitizer for 20 seconds. It's more of a 5-second slapping motion. I think standing outside a patient's room for 20 seconds would be perceived as too long for a nurse. (So much to do, so little time). All the media talk has been on soap and water hand-washing. Even the auditors didn't care how long it took. I know better now.

I remember calling hand sanitizers antiseptic or antibacterial alcohol gels. Isopropyl (or ethyl) alcohol is the crucial active ingredient. So, I never noticed when over-the-counter hand sanitizers started to claim to be anti-microbial and "99.9% effective against germs." I never used any prior to working in a hospital. Instead, I opted for soap and water.

Meanwhile, out in the community, the variety of hand sanitizers and their use exploded since COVID-19. Product shortages and overcharging ensued for a while (Sophia Harris, "Customers complain of price gouging as hand sanitizer sells out in stores," March 2020). It looked like every store had a hand dispenser near their entrance. Some businesses had ones that really stunk or were too drippy.

I preferred the ones in the hospital, except that the skin on my hands is always very dry from its mandatory and frequent use. Perhaps that's why nurses prefer soap and water, which can be considered a mini spa treatment in comparison. As a result, dry hands had become an occupational reality.

CHAPTER 20

Screening Patients Daily

With the advent of COVID-19, everyone was screened as of March 2020. Screening started at the entrance to the hospital. The password to get in was "No" to all screening questions. In the beginning, the list of questions included recent travel to China. The list kept getting longer with the discovery and addition of more symptoms.

The poor screeners tried to ask these questions in the beginning. Shortly thereafter, the questions were posted instead. Not sure if they were posted outside the hospital at any point. But once plexiglass barriers were in place (to protect the screener), the sheet of questions was taped on it. Pedestrian traffic still caused lineups, especially with social distancing.

A brilliant idea was the screening app for staff at my hospital. It eliminated most of the crowd at the back entrance. This was especially important as some people wouldn't put on a mask until they were inside the building. With the app one could review the current screening questions and obtain a green pass. Staff showed this green screen to gain entry.

Traffic at the doors eased as staff were fast-tracked inside. One still had to show a work ID badge. I don't know why some employees hesitated to do so. Your length of employment had no bearing. If you are returning from the previous day, no difference. It's just rude being noncompliant at this very basic level of security, and a hassle for the screeners.

The entrance protocol became: show ID badge and green pass on your smartphone, wash hands with sanitizer, and get a new face mask from the screener. Then you're in, but the nurse is not done until arriving at her/his unit.

As of July 2022, the paid screeners were let go, and the hospital moved to a passive screening system. This was in response to provincial guidelines. Now the public can access an online screening questionnaire which includes a question about being fully vaccinated. So, the last answer now should be "Yes."

In the second year of COVID-19 (2021) we started screening all inpatients. This may have been a response to continued outbreaks in nursing units. Outbreaks were declared if two patients got infected, but this was now redefined as one or two people as per the new provincial guidelines. The units with outbreaks were now publicized on the hospital's website.

Nurses read the screening questions daily to patients to see if they had developed any new symptoms while in hospital. The symptom list, by November 2020, was: "fever, chills, headache, cough, shortness of breath, sore throat or difficulty swallowing, runny nose or congestion with no other cause, loss of taste or smell, arthralgia (joint pain), myalgia (muscle pain), eye pain or conjunctivitis, nausea or vomiting, diarrhea, abdominal pain, unusual fatigue, lethargy or malaise, unexplained fall, decreased level of consciousness or delirium, and unexplained worsening of a chronic condition."

The patients got tired of this, but occasionally someone answered "Yes." Then it was the question of whether to swab the patient. Technically, if swabbing a suspected COVID-19 patient, the patient also needs to be isolated in a private room.

Nurses can order certain tests like the COVID-19 NP swabs without a doctor's order. We were used to this with suspected C-difficile, which already required immediate isolation until test results were returned. So, it became even more important that there was enough suspicion to even do the test before it became a logistical problem.

For many years now, our hospital has been running at full capacity. Even at night the Administrator-on-Call (night nursing supervisor) would fill up any bed and assume there would be discharges the following morning to allow for any new arrivals. This caused a lot of tension between the nurses and nursing management.

Pre-COVID the lack of flexible beds also led to hallway patients. But you can't have patients in the hallway during COVID-19. The risk is too high, whether from airborne or droplet transmission. So, suddenly moving patients from room to room to accommodate an "isolation" patient became more frequent. A headache for the Charge Nurse for sure, and those helping to move furniture.

Luckily, all the surgical patients and patients with epilepsy were tested upon admission. Surgical patients needed testing to reduce unknown post-operative complications and to maintain the standard sterility of the operating room. Meanwhile, patients admitted to have EEG monitoring needed scalp electrodes to be applied, and had to be tested to safeguard the technicians who were in close body proximity during the procedure. Also, the electrodes could potentially be cross contaminated between patients. However, all other patients were only screened.

Symptoms can take several days to show up if they ever do. I think this is where the hospital should've done better. All admitted patients should have been tested for COVID-19. This is especially important as hospitals accept unvaccinated and vaccinated patients alike. The use of the precautionary principle didn't go far enough.

A hard truth is that people fudge their screening answers as we're basing this on the *honour system.* We expect you to answer truthfully or to the best of your knowledge. I believe objective data, like testing, is more expensive but is far more reliable than subjective answers.

I think the hospital executives, or the provincial government, had decided not to test every patient. Maybe no hospital in the world does. Google can't tell me. Perhaps only a small island nation can. It's not cost-effective until proven.

Screening, on the other hand, is a relatively inexpensive alternative. A first cautionary step perhaps, but not precautionary enough. It's not what the SARS Commission meant with the precautionary principle: "Where there is reasonable evidence of an impending threat to public harm, it is inappropriate to require proof of causation beyond reasonable doubt before taking steps to avert the threat ... that reasonable efforts to reduce risk need not await scientific proof." (Justice Campbell, 2006).

Nurses were to screen all patients twice a day. I don't think anyone did. I tried to incorporate it into my morning assessment. Often patients remarked no one asked them these questions in several days. I had no response to this, but we were all very busy all the time. Alas, I can only be responsible for my own actions.

I remember moving symptomatic patients into private rooms. Sometimes we would bump private coverage patients out of their rooms to do this. Isolation precautions overrode the opportunity to generate private room income.

If the NP swab came back negative, the patient would be moved back, if possible. Relocating a patient is a two-person job. There's a lot of work involved moving beds and tables. Nurses do this. Sometimes the PCAs or Ward Clerk would help. Housekeeping had to do a terminal clean of the temporary isolation room too.

This task of moving beds wasn't mentioned in nursing school. I remember in various job descriptions, where the last line always stated, "and other responsibilities, as assigned and/or requested" (i.e., help whenever needed). I think I saw that line in my job description at CIBC too. But it seems to me that nurses are always doing more of the last line than what we were hired for. We wear many hats.

CHAPTER 21

COVID-19 Research

Research matters. I find it very ironic that a COVID-19 research study was called "RESPECT." The very thing nurses have been wanting for ages but crystallized when the Ontario government's Bill 124 expressed a deliberate show of *disrespect* (i.e., wage suppression in union contracts). Now respect was being used in a different way. I guess the universe has a strange sense of humour.

When I heard of this study's name, I had to scratch my head. It did not compute. The study's acronym spelled out is: **Re**search Platform to **S**creen and **Prot**ect Health care Workers. It began in March 2020, but I enrolled in the study April 28, 2020. Then I re-enrolled July 16, 2020, for the RESPECT 2 Study, when it was then expanded to include food industry workers.

I have been a participant in countless studies over the years. What better way to learn about your body and its health status without having to be sick first? So, it was a no-brainer to enroll. Also, it gave me some confidence to know (with objective data) that I wasn't spreading COVID-19 to anyone, including my own patients or family.

The eligibility criteria for the initial RESPECT Study were to be a health care worker at University Health Network (UHN) and be asymptomatic. It was also convenient as there was onsite testing. Plus, one could be tested as frequently as once a week, but that got old very quickly. The nasal swab (NP swab) hurt more than the blood test. Maybe my nares are more sensitive due to my history of sinusitis.

The main test would be done by polymerase chain reaction (PCR) test via a NP swab. Later, bloodwork was added for past or current exposure to infection, or active infection itself. In April 2021, when vaccines were available, the researchers were able to add the blood test for COVID-19 vaccine antibody levels.

Of course, one was screened to be tested as asymptomatic. Symptoms are subjective. COVID-19 symptoms are similar to regular colds, coughs, and sore throats. It took a discerning person to recognize if they were experiencing something unusual for them.

When loss of smell was added to the growing list of known COVID-19 symptoms I had to reconsider my own reduced sense of smell and taste. However, I had these deficits prior to the pandemic. Therefore, it was a matter of determining if they were getting worse due to COVID-19, wearing a face mask at work, or the aging process. It's still an ongoing issue for me.

I was very excited once the researchers added the antibody level blood test and had ten of these done throughout the study. I saw a pattern of numbers rising towards 9,000, then declining, but never back down to the original low of 135. I was happy. Vaccines had raised the antibody count, as promised, and I had not contracted COVID-19 yet.

Could I have been a COVID-19 unicorn? Resistance is not futile in this context. I have heard the term *Novid* on *CBC News Explore's* "About That" program with Andrew Chang (February 2, 2023). This designation refers to people who have never caught COVID-19. The current reasons for this phenomenon include: always taking precautions, having a natural resistance, or just thinking they've never been infected (i.e., asymptomatic), but were. Not a lot of research or media coverage has been devoted to this aspect of the pandemic experience. I prefer option one—having taken precautions.

I continue to be annoyed by how the media and other commentators kept harping on about how vaccines didn't keep the antibody levels high.

No one has come out with a consensus of what the COVID-19 antibody range should be. There might be ranges for other vaccines, but I have never heard of them either. There are antibody titer tests for other diseases like hepatitis, chickenpox, rabies, measles, mumps, rubella, and TB. The test results are either positive or negative. So why are we expecting more from the COVID-19 antibody titer tests?

The Ontario Health Study also did antibody tests for its participants. However, they acknowledged upfront the test results did not confirm COVID-19 infection, only the presence of antibodies in response to infection or vaccination. I do not see how this was useful information for anyone. My results were positive both times. I had been vaccinated. This did not give me any comfort, confidence, or knowledge. Why didn't they use the same blood test as the RESPECT 2 Study?

The RESPECT Studies had useful findings. They found that 0.5% of the asymptomatic health care workers who were swabbed were COVID-19 positive. Meanwhile, in the RESPECT 2 Study, antibody tests revealed 1.4–3.4% asymptomatic workers were infected. I didn't hear the media jump on this. To me, this means even while using PPE health care workers are at risk at work or elsewhere. Plus, HCWs could be taking unknown chances and spreading the virus when not masked in public places.

I was very unhappy when the RESPECT 2 Study closed. I guess they reached the study's objective. But I no longer had a way to get tested as an asymptomatic person, except by using the home kits.

The Rapid Antigen Tests (RATs) that are freely available in Ontario are problematic for me. I got my first test kit after waiting two hours in line at a shopping mall, and now my grocery store has them at checkout. Everyone acknowledges that they are less accurate than PCR and prone to false negative results (Christopher Labos, "Navigating False Negatives on COVID-19 Rapid Tests," April 2022). Plus, there are so many ways to do the tests incorrectly on oneself. At least with the RESPECT Studies or at a COVID-19 Assessment Centre, I knew it was being done properly. I didn't trust myself since my nostrils are sensitive and the swab always hurts.

CHAPTER 22

Looming Chaos

Chaos theory suggests there is a pattern in the disorganized events we observe or experience. We just need to see the bigger picture, not the individual crises or changes. Most of the time we are amid chaos and can't see anything ahead, above, below, or around ourselves.

In 2006 I wrote a university paper on chaos theory and nursing leadership, concluding it was an opportunity for growth, creativity, and resilience. Little did I know, decades later, I would see no real opportunity for nursing leadership in the workplace, except in the nurses' union. Instead, I would witness chaos theory and corporate/political leadership up close and personal during COVID-19.

The Ontario government did not adapt as quickly as it could to the pandemic and has now decided, after two years, that the crisis is over despite the Chief Medical Officer of Health Dr. Kieran Moore, saying otherwise. Headlines have included: "Ontario to drop most mask mandates on March 21, remaining pandemic rules to be lifted by end of April" (*CBC News,*

March 9, 2022), and "Ontario Progressive Conservatives campaigning as if COVID-19 pandemic is over, experts say" (Holly McKenzie-Sutter, *The Canadian Press*, April 24, 2022). In that same first article by Sara Jabakhanji and Julia Knope, they quoted Dr. Moore as saying, "removing the mask mandate 'does not mean the risk is gone' or the pandemic is over." Then, another striking headline appeared: "7th wave of COVID-19 rising across the province, Public Health Ontario's latest report says" (*CBC News*, July 14, 2022). The government's focus had moved from masks to vaccines. The pandemic continues.

I believe hospital leadership did a much better job of adapting and continues to do so. The safety of patients and the vulnerable in the community should be an ongoing concern as we move into the future.

Hospitals have been the epicentre of the COVID-19 pandemic. The hardest hit areas were the ICU and ED units. I was in another unit but also severely stressed, nonetheless. The domino effect in action.

The first time I wrote about COVID-19 in my journal was February 10, 2020. I wasn't yet concerned as few people in Ontario had been infected with the new coronavirus.

I had other things on my mind. My sister had moved in with me in October 2019, and I had a family christening coming up in Calgary. I did go to Calgary, but I was masked whenever I could. I've had experience with roommates before. It never lasts long. Living with someone else is stressful even if you think you know them. Within a short while of my sister living with me, I developed a shingles-like rash on my neck.

I also started worrying about money and decided to cancel my cable TV. I was advised by younger colleagues that cable was so passé. Netflix, Crave, and YouTube were in. So, no more instant news updates on the CP24 channel. I had to hunt for my COVID-19 news.

On February 14, 2020, the hospital where I worked had the Infection, Prevention and Control (IPAC) department monitoring the COVID-19 situation and screening staff for travel to China. I had been on a trip to China myself in 2018 (my last big trip abroad before focusing on the rest of Canada). I assumed everyone in a communist country would wear black or white clothing. Wrong. Most young adults were very fashionable. I also noticed how the cities are crowded and work differently, something that's not surprising given China's 1.4 billion population. It's why they have massive traffic jams at every major city intersection, and lineups are ubiquitous.

A nurse from China had suggested taking a face mask, I assumed for the air pollution (and I packed some), but my sinuses and nostrils were so congested from the airplane's recirculating air that I didn't feel the need to use one. Was this a foreshadowing of things to come?

Everyone thought this COVID-19 would fade away like a receding wave. They didn't think it was another SARS despite eventually calling the virus SARS-CoV-2 (Severe Acute Respiratory Syndrome Coronavirus 2). At first, they called it just the *Novel Coronavirus* (a placeholder name). Coronavirus is one of the family of viruses of the common cold. It didn't sound dangerous.

To be fair, most of the incoming information was being collected and analyzed as quickly as possible by the WHO, their established partners in research and policy, and other reliable sources. And just like SARS, this virus had originated in China, but in Wuhan, in the province of Hubei.

By March 13, 2020, news broke out about the Canadian prime minister's wife, Sophie Grégoire, who had been infected while in London, UK. It sounded like this virus wasn't going away, but escalating. It finally felt real and potentially dangerous. I started watching the WHO COVID-19 updates on YouTube. The WHO had already declared COVID-19 a pandemic on March 11, 2020. Later, I found that the Johns Hopkins University (JHU) website was better, as it listed the daily COVID-19 cases and deaths of each country. For once I was glad Canada was not in the top 10 of a list.

CHAPTER 23

Hospital Leadership

I have to say my hospital leadership did much better than their provincial counterpart. Frequent communication and COVID-19 updates were facilitated via Zoom-like meetings that were streamed and later accessible. This was in addition to unit managers' morning meetings.

This forum allowed for staff to ask questions, bring awareness about certain concerns, and give a sense of *we were all in this together.* I felt we were a community with townhall meetings every week, then every two weeks for the first two years of COVID-19.

As a result of the staff's concern about the supply of PPE, the levels of supplies were posted on the staff website. When the amount of COVID-19 infected patients was known, but not of infected staff, that was added as well. This was information staff needed to assess their own risk level, not to satisfy curiosity.

I also submitted a question: Why weren't we in a Code Orange situation? When this code was initially introduced, it described protocols to follow if a mass event occurred outside the hospital. Shouldn't a pandemic count? I think the annually updated Disaster Plan Fan-Out for each unit was part of this preparation. It was a telephone tree of who calls whom and for all available staff to come to work. The Code Orange example given was SARS. So, I had this stuck in my head for years.

Alas, my question was never answered. Forum questions had to be provided ahead of the scheduled meeting and were rated by how many people agreed this was a worthy or popular question. I don't know how this part worked, but it must've been a different app or website. I certainly never voted on the forum questions.

It was later that I noticed that Code Orange was primarily described as mass casualties outside the hospital from one incident. I guess this referred to acute injuries from a traffic accident or building collapse. I know that when there was an expected high influx of protesters or festival attendees in the city, the hospital would be on high alert. But we weren't a trauma hospital. We wouldn't be anyone's first choice, unless maybe for the overflow of injured people.

I now understood Code Orange had morphed into a high emergency that would last until the last patient was treated from that single mass casualty incident or disaster. My hospital had also participated in a mock Code Orange exercise in December 2019 where this was the case. It was prescient—my hospital would use parts of its disaster plan for COVID-19.

Looking back to SARS, the Ontario government had ordered all GTA hospitals to activate their Code Orange plans March 26, 2003 (Donald E. Low, *SARS: Lessons from Toronto*, 2004). If SARS was indeed a Code Orange, why wasn't this the case for COVID-19 at my hospital?

In January 2022 it was reported that two hospitals issued Code Oranges. William Osler Health System (Etobicoke General & Brampton Civic hospitals) said their nurse-to-patient ratio had climbed from over 1:4 to almost 1:10. I can't imagine the stress on those nurses, or the scared patients. Even under normal circumstances, 1:5 is a big ask.

The other hospital, Queensway Carleton, in Ottawa, had also rung the Code Orange bell. So, I'm still confused. Maybe this is the hospital's version of a state of emergency where more resources suddenly become available. Maybe my hospital was better prepared this time.

COVID-19 is not a single event—one and done. It's a series of events captured as COVID waves. It's the virus that keeps on giving. It will keep going on and on. Three years of COVID-19 hospital protocols so far. It's become the new normal as Ontario has accumulated 1.6 million cases of COVID-19 infected people, and 16,729 deaths (Public Health Ontario, August 5, 2023). That's a thousand more deaths since January 2023—a mere seven months earlier. And new COVID-19 variants are on the horizon.

CHAPTER 24

Good Decisions

My hospital made some excellent choices and adaptations that showed leadership, creativity, and growth. The hospital administration let the IPAC manager lead with many COVID-19 related changes and innovations. I was amazed at all the following adaptations that were required for a hospital in pandemic mode:

- Restricted access to the hospital included screeners (like sentries) at entrances. Sometimes it would be security staff. Everyone was screened and had to wear a face mask upon entry.
- Reduced visitors from no limit 24/7 access to one designated essential care partner (or alternate) per day. The nursing care model is the *patient-centred care model.* It recognizes that family and friends are important to the emotional wellbeing of patients. We always assume this to be a positive relationship and helpful to the nurse caring for the patient.

- The hospital's food court seating was closed, but counter service of various restaurants remained open. Staff relied on large amounts of coffee and tea to keep going. It was also time consuming to leave the hospital for outside food. My staff lounge had limited seating. Sometimes I ate in my locker room.

- As previously mentioned, great innovations were the forum for COVID-19 updates and questions, COVID-19 dedicated websites, a staff screening app, and the transparency of PPE supplies. It was a great idea to provide a variety of eye protection of full-face shields, goggles, and hybrid face masks.

- A designated COVID-19 unit, not ICU, but for stable infected patients that required 1:2 nurse-to-patient care. Meanwhile, other units decreased their patient censuses where possible. Elective surgeries were cancelled.

- Code Blue was now an enhanced version called *Protected Code Blue*. It meant that CPR was recognized to possibly generate aerosols, and all code team members were to wear full airborne PPE during the code. (Code Blues in hospitals, by the way, don't involve mouth-to-mouth resuscitation). The Code Blue cart had extra devices including a Tavish® respirator for the patient during transport to ICU.

- A COVID-19 Assessment Centre was set up in a vacant bank building nearby. Occupational Health was no longer seeing employees without advance notice. The assessment centre was for staff and the public who had COVID-like symptoms or had exposures to infected patients.

- The RESPECT Study (previously discussed in Chapter 21), which began early in the pandemic, was a great opportunity for asymptomatic employees to get tested. A win-win situation.

- Voluntary redeployment of staff to long-term care facilities when the need was greatest. Also much later, redeployed office staff to nursing units as "patient assistants."

- Increased level of cleaning of all touchable services and the one-time air duct cleaning.

- Mandatory vaccinations for all hospital staff. If the idea of a hospital is that it is open to all patients (even infected ones), then the staff needs to be vigilant in protecting all patients and fellow workers. A hospital should be a protective health bubble.

- Once vaccines were available, vaccine invites were sent via staff email. Mass vaccinations were done at the MaRS Centre. There were other options open to staff if recorded by the Ontario COVID-19 Proof of Vaccination document. Staff had to later send this information to Occupational Health.

- A COVID-19 Respite room dedicated for staff to relax away from their unit. It was a quiet space that had snacks. Unfortunately, I rarely had the opportunity to use it.

- Free parking for staff was donated by the hospital's Board of Trustees (and/or the hospital's foundation). It lasted only a few months but was very appreciated at the time.

- Advocating for all hospital staff to get the provincial government's Temporary Pandemic Pay. Physiotherapists and occupational therapists were notably excluded.

- A hospital sabbatical program called "Post-COVID Pause." They should have called it "Mid-COVID Pause," as there was no post-COVID yet in 2021. The benefit offered days up to a month away from work. It was time off without pay, extra vacation time that had to be pre-approved by your manager. I really looked forward to this. However, after my month off I felt like I had never left.

- Unlike some hospitals, my regular vacation was never cancelled. However, my vacation only meant I could sleep in. Travel was restricted or still unsafe. The pandemic was still with us.

The chaos of COVID-19 had created opportunities for hospital leadership to develop a variety of initiatives that were practical, but also showed care for its workers and patients. I was impressed.

CHAPTER 25

Other Decisions

There were other decisions my hospital made that I didn't agree with. No one asked for input from nurses, as far as I know. The talk about resilience and mental health was superficial for me. I've listed these decisions using bullet points:

- Mandatory redeployment of nurses. An example was redeploying staff to ICU for a day. That was so stressful and useless. The ICU nurse had a second pair of hands, but the temporary nurse didn't know where certain supplies were kept (without any orientation to the unit) or how things were done differently there.

My ICU nurse had her patient transferred to a level-2 bed, so we ended up with two then three patients. She asked me for a Doppler ultrasound device I couldn't find (it was locked away in a cupboard). Another patient required a blood transfusion, for which the new protocol was to use an IV pump. She was still using IV by gravity and then the patient's vein blew. I felt like it was my fault.

Why did ICU nurses need regular RNs to help them? I thought, at the very least, I would be doing VS and neuro assessments every hour. No. The bedside cardiac monitors attached to the patients read all the vitals including respirations. The one patient I did recognize from my unit never had a neuro assessment done in my presence at all. I don't remember his diagnosis. Maybe he was a neurology patient who didn't speak English? I still don't know what expertise I was providing, if any.

I ended up watching all three patients as a Constant Observer by the end of the shift. Two of them had mitts on to prevent pulling on an external ventricular drain or the transfusion line, and the last patient was just confused and restless. They were on opposite sides of the pod hallway, so I felt like I was a hockey goalie again, frequently checking left and right.

We were given an ICU resource manual prior to going there, but it didn't address these situations. This was simply temporary redeployment of nurses by management.

I did see an ICU nurse with a COVID-19 patient down the hallway in another pod. I could tell because there were a lot of yellow-gown people in the room to help her. She was directing them like a queen.

We were also redeployed to another unit for two days or a week. Each unit has a specialty, so unless I had neurology or neurosurgery patients, I was out of my comfort zone again. However, the nurses there were much nicer and welcoming. This time we had our own patients.

- Even though we had reduced patients on our unit, and therefore fewer nurses, the night nursing supervisor would continue to push new or transfer patients.
- Since elective surgeries have restarted, the patient census is back to pre-COVID levels. The concept of operating beds at full capacity is still a dilemma. It allows for no flexibility when the unexpected need for a bed arises (e.g., emergency transfers, admissions, or isolation requirements).

- We should have used N95 masks right from the start like we did for SARS. It seems incongruent that nurses had to be mask fitted every two years for N95 masks only to be told not to use them during a respiratory pandemic. I suspect provincial interference. I also never knew these masks expired.
- All admitted patients should have been tested for COVID-19, not just the surgical or epilepsy unit patients. All should have been considered at risk for contracting the virus.
- Lastly, we should have stayed with one visitor per day (not the current two). We should not attempt to return to the pre-COVID visitors' policy. The hospital environment has changed. If staff must use antiviral equipment and be vaccinated, why are visitors less protected and patients even less so? It doesn't sound like we are all in this together anymore, or that this is the most protected environment it could be.

There are probably good reasons for these decisions that I was not privy to. Some decisions seemed like good optics (i.e., good in theory, but not in practice). I sense political mandates or concerns were involved.

However, despite other unknown factors impacting these decisions, I still believe we should have tested every patient for the virus. It would have been the right step. Prevention begins with monitoring and testing. Screening wasn't enough for patient safety or patient care. The bar for hospitals should have been higher for at-risk people.

CHAPTER 26

Hospital as a Fortress

If the hospital became a "fortress" then nurses were the HCW warriors inside the fortress walls. Nurses had armour to protect them from the viral enemy. The uniforms remained the same, but PPE like face masks, face shields, and scrub caps were added. As soon as vaccines were available, the vaccine became another layer of protection, but on the inside of the body.

However, 46 Canadian health care workers still died as of January 2022, according to the Canadian Institute for Health Information's (CIHI's) fourth and final iteration of "COVID-19 cases and death in health care workers in Canada" (CIHI, March 31, 2022). SARS (2003) as I mentioned before, had three official HCW deaths under very different circumstances.

The concept of HCWs as warriors or soldiers is repeated in the following heartfelt expression of respect and gratitude from Jian Xiao et al in "SARS, MERS and COVID-19 among healthcare workers: A narrative review", *Journal of Infection and Public Health*, 2020. The article concludes with "… HCWs are soldiers. Their enemies are viruses and they fight the wars without gun smoke…Although, in the face of the epidemic, they are [sic] may also be worried, afraid, and anxious. However, because of the responsibility, as long as the situation needs, HCWs rush to the battlefield without hesitation. We pay tribute to frontline fighting HCWs, thank them for their great efforts."

Instead of a soldier's helmet, nurses have a voluntary scrub cap. The current scrub caps are not a sentimental return to the nurse's white hat or cap. Those were discontinued (1980s and 1990s) because they were full of bacteria and were not washable. Meanwhile, the white uniform changed to scrubs due to fashion trends and more male nurses entering the field. Today's washable scrub cap is optional and worn to protect nurses' hair from COVID-19. For others, like me, the buttons on the side of the caps protect the nurses' ears from the ear loops of face masks.

I recall a stranger came to our unit and offered free homemade scrub caps. She carried a bag and asked us to choose one or two. I chose a yellow one with a subtle wheat design. The other one had bright flowers on a black background. I found out later other nursing communities had similar experiences of community donations (e.g., Vancouver Island, April 2020).

At the beginning of COVID-19 the media and the public called all frontline health care workers *warriors*. This acknowledged the dangerous and essential work people like nurses did. We were recognized as being brave and worthy. They honoured us at the hospital with free meals and other gifts. This kept our spirits up to continue the good fight.

In the community we were also appreciated. In the College and Bathurst neighbourhood some residents banged pots at 7:00 p.m. outside their homes. As I drove on Palmerston Blvd. one evening, I heard some noise and turned towards it. I realized what it meant when I saw two neighbours with pots on their front porch. It made me cry to realize that this rumour was a real phenomenon in Toronto. I stopped my car and thanked them in return. They made "noise" to acknowledge HCWs' contributions. This was heartfelt on both sides.

Some businesses also gave free coffee to HCWs with ID badges or allowed them to jump the long line-ups to get inside Walmart. I was embarrassed to jump the line, but I did ask for a free coffee once at a drive-thru Starbucks with my badge.

As the pandemic continued this privilege has stopped. No more *scarcity buying* for toilet paper or antimicrobial cleaners. The public was tired and had moved on to other priorities, but the nurses who remain working in the hospitals have not moved on. They still need your support and recognition. Nurses still wear the anti-viral shields— face masks and face shields or goggles.

Wearing pandemic gear all the time at work was isolating. Sometimes I couldn't tell people apart and had to guess by body shape alone. The ID badges on lanyards were rarely facing forward. And while wearing the masks and face shields, talking became an effort. Being in the staff lounge was a treat until it wasn't. It became restricted to safe seating for 6 people. I would eat lunch at my locker when the max amount of people was already there. I felt even more alone at work than before.

Ironic because I like my solitude outside of work. I'm an introvert but do like a tiny bit of socialization. Interactions with coworkers provided friendships and moral support. It never occurred to me to phone or text a coworker during this time. I needed this social contact at work to energize me to do the relentless work of nursing.

As a result of my reduced communication, I didn't know how other coworkers were coping. In the early days of COVID-19 I heard of a nurse, who would remove her uniform in her garage, then shower before any contact with her family. I wasn't doing that. I only had my sister living with me then.

I tried to follow the hospital rules. I would put on my uniform at work and remove it in the locker room. After a year I only changed my scrub top there. I was tired before I even got to my unit to start my shift. The fatigue was incremental, just like the frog in a slow boiling pot. Another "rule" was to change one's mask twice per shift. This one I just forgot to do, or the effort was too much at the time.

The hospital is no longer a fortress if it ever truly was one during this pandemic. More access has been given recently to visitors. The nurses are no longer as protected as they once were. With the increase to two essential care partners per patient, the level of risk is increased as well. The circle of care has expanded and so has the danger. The discontinuation of active screening has made it easier to lie to a computer than to a person.

Outbreaks of COVID-19 on nursing units continue in 2023, becoming the norm. I'm not saying who caused these outbreaks, but the increased foot traffic and opportunity for the virus to spread remain.

There were two outbreaks on my unit while I was there. The first one was in March 2020. I think it was a transferred patient from a stepdown unit, where the original outbreak was discovered. The next was in January 2022. This patient was a new admission. I don't recall if he was tested or just screened. Luckily, I was not infected, and was absent during the subsequent isolation of patients and terminal cleaning procedures. It was during my Post-COVID Pause break.

In the spring of 2022, I admitted a surgical patient who declined to be tested for COVID-19. He said he tested himself (with RAT) and he hadn't gone outside his home for several days. I reiterated he can't go to surgery without a PCR test, and home tests don't count.

In fact, we have no way to indicate home test results in our computer system. I think positive RAT tests should be noted somewhere. This is another example of the honour system. We rely heavily on patients' self-disclosure for medication and past medical histories.

Even though there is no spot on the Pre-Op Checklist, I always tried to include the date of the NP swab test and result. Plus, the headache from any preventable delay to surgeries was to be avoided at all costs.

The patient finally relented after I continued the admission process and returned to advocating the required test. It turns out he was, in fact, positive and was sent home to recover and self-isolate. He had no symptoms. We were both shocked.

I miss the 2003 SARS protocols. There were no outbreaks at my hospital back then because each patient was treated as if they were already infected. Every patient room was an isolation room. N95 masks ruled the day. No visitors were allowed, except for families of dying patients. I have no idea if my hospital had a SARS patient, but I felt safer back then.

With today's technology visiting can be done via FaceTime or Google Duo (now known as Google Meet). However, the patient's nurse should not be the one setting this up. Perhaps a hospital volunteer? There is only one tablet (on a pole with wheels) on our unit that can be cleaned and used for this purpose. Perhaps patients can use their own tablets or cellphones, and families can take this on.

If patients stayed a shorter time in hospital this wouldn't be needed at all. But patients are staying longer due to a variety of reasons, including complications due to surgery, and poor life planning about where to go next, if home isn't safe anymore. Families should have these difficult talks before a loved one ends up in hospital. I would suggest the hospital isn't as safe either … for the patient, the visitor, or for the nurse.

CHAPTER 27

COVID-19 Waves

COVID's Wave 1 created global chaos with numerous images of anxiety, suffering, and death in so many countries. I was glued to the television to watch the federal and provincial updates on COVID-19. It was "must-see TV" as new updates happened weekly. Nurses were working hard inside the hospitals, but what was happening outside of them?

The COVID-19 waves of infected cases kept coming. To the best of my knowledge, these were the Ontario waves (slightly different for Canada as a whole): Wave 1: February 2020 to August 2020; Wave 2: September 2020 to mid-February 2021; Wave 3: mid-February 2021 to June 2021; Wave 4: September 2021 to November 2021; Wave 5: December 2021 to February 2022; Wave 6: March 2022 to May 2022; Wave 7: July 2022 to August 2022; Wave 8: September 2022 to November 2022. We are probably in Wave 9 in January 2023. But who's admitting to this? The government and media stopped publicly discussing COVID waves after Wave 4.

On January 15, 2020, the federal government opened its Emergency Operations Centre (EOC). On January 25, 2020, our first COVID-19 case was confirmed, and it was travel related. On March 18, 2020, the capacity of lab testing had to be increased. The following day, on March 19, 2020, the federal government announced 96 research projects focused on "development and implementation measures to detect, manage and reduce transmission of COVID-19."

We were introduced to Dr. Theresa Tam on March 23, 2020, when she started public service announcements on television and radio. The first message was about handwashing, social distancing, and against unnecessary travel. Later, it would include non-medical face masks in public. By November 3, 2020, Public Health started endorsing the three-layer, non-medical masks.

She advised us in April 2020 that 50% of the COVID-19 infected, and 79% of the deaths were in long-term care (LTC) facilities. The new recommendations were to restrict visitors and volunteers, prevent workers from working at more than one location, the use of PPE, physical distancing, and screening staff and essential visitors.

The federal government offered the Canadian Armed Forces to the provinces and territories to assist with the crisis in LTC. Only Ontario and Québec accepted this help. My hospital also offered volunteers, and a nurse on my unit participated at a LTC facility for a month.

In the first COVID-19 wave most of the cases were community related after the initial travel-related ones. States of Emergency were eventually declared by all provinces and territories. The city of Toronto also called on a State of Emergency that would last 777 days, whereas the province of Ontario would declare and end its State of Emergency several times.

I wasn't scared. I lived through the SARS experience in the hospital. I expected something similar, but I was wrong. COVID-19 wasn't just in the hospital but everywhere this time.

Perhaps this was the scariest time for others as we had no vaccine yet, and we had no idea how long the virus would take to burn itself out. Lockdowns and stay-at-home orders were declared.

I had a letter from my employer confirming I was an essential worker should I get stopped driving on the deserted streets. However, the definition of an essential worker kept growing. At one point, the media confirmed dog walkers were added, and I felt insulted that nurses were as essential as them. Why weren't the dog owners walking their own pets? A First World problem or situation, for sure. I'm hoping I'll laugh at this eventually, but not yet.

CHAPTER 28

Ontario's Bill 124 and Nurses

Nurses are essential workers, yet the provincial government didn't treat us with any respect before the pandemic. Then when COVID-19 hit, this government was scrambling to patch up their mistakes without acknowledging any wrongdoing. Selective memory, indeed.

The Ontario government had been a mess during COVID-19, but it just reflected this government's mind set. "Tax cuts" are the perennial Conservative party's slogan and solution. But taxes pay for public nurses, teachers, and other provincial employees. Bill 124 was the tool to legitimize wage suppression for provincial public employees, which was to ensure a better future for generations to come. Instead, the bill hurt the very people you would depend on during the pandemic or any life-or-death emergency.

What is Bill 124? In November 2019 "Protecting a Sustainable Public Sector for Future Generations Act" came into effect and was made retroactive to June 5, 2019. It was thought to be a smart idea by the Ontario Conservative government. Their mantra has always been tax cuts (and negative election campaigns). But aren't governments supposed to provide social support to taxpayers, including their public service employees? Taxes are the traditional way to finance collective needs such as health care, education, and police. Yet, here we see a smokescreen of selective accounting and selective targets.

Provincial public sector jobs include the fields of municipal or provincial government, protective services, education, community services, and health care. Yet exceptions were made. The municipal police, doctors, and firefighters were excluded from this bill. The Ontario Provincial Police (OPP) were included but their contracts were four years long and were not affected yet. The remaining public sectors, like those of nurses, had salaries capped to 1% for three years (the moderation period).

The provincial government had substantially interfered with the Ontario Nurses' Association's (ONA's) ability to negotiate a fair union contract. It was as if there was no arbitrator present at all, with the Ontario government acting like a third party, but with all the power. There was no real negotiating in good faith.

Was this a gender-focused target or simply a numbers strategy? The excluded professions from the bill were mostly male-dominated jobs. Nursing is mainly female dominated, with only 9% male nurses. Also, there are 31,500 doctors and 26,100 police officers in Ontario, while there are 117,102 nurses who were affected. It seems like obvious discrimination, even if it was an unconscious or systemic bias.

Months after Bill 124 became law the first COVID-19 patient arrived at Sunnybrook Hospital (Toronto) in January 2020. Two years later we had more than a million COVID-19 cases. Three years later we have 4.6 million infected people (cases) in Canada in a population of 39 million. Ontario is not providing this data anymore. All I can find are bar graphs of wastewater surveillance.

Public schools were closed March 12, 2020, transitioning to remote/distance learning with heavy reliance on the parents to pick up the slack. Nurses are parents too. Luckily, some have extended families to help. It's not just babysitting but learning "the new math" or science. Everyone now had to have a computer at home as well.

At least four States of Emergency were called: March 17, 2020 to July 24, 2020; January 12, 2021 to February 10, 2021; April 8, 2021 to June 2, 2021; and February 11, 2022 to February 23, 2022. The last one should have been embarrassing as the prime minister had to invoke the Emergencies Act to resolve the "anti-COVID-19 mandate" protesters' occupation of Ottawa, so the province finally acquiesced to some action. Too little, too late.

During Wave 1 the pandemic exposed the sad state of the LTC facilities and its residents. During Wave 3 the high ICU patient count in hospitals was extreme. Nurses were leaving after being overworked, and suffering from burnout and disrespect. The provincial government was responsible. Bill 124 was overturned by Justice Koehnen on November 29, 2022, but Premier Ford appealed the decision, while claiming to love nurses (March 2023). Still insisting on saving money … on the backs of unionized nurses.

COVID's Wave 5 got lost in the provincial updates. I recall France announcing Wave 5 had arrived, but it was all quiet here in Ontario, with no announcement or reference, and no updates to modelling (a tool for predicting the future course of the spread of COVID-19). Meanwhile, infected cases were the highest due to the arrival of the Omicron variant. Was this when testing via PCR swabs became too much for the labs and we began relying on wastewater surveillance? Now we rely on stats based on community wastewater for indicators of the SARS-CoV-2 virus from anonymously infected people.

The problem is twofold. Asymptomatic infected people who were contagious would not know they should use the home test kit, and therefore, would not self-isolate or use a face mask. Plus, how would Public Health alert them? Forget contact tracing. The wastewater doesn't indicate who is infected, only the larger community where they reside or work. So, our case counts are not accurate or personally useful. As a result, we are underreporting our COVID-19 case counts.

How is this data collection better than PCR testing (via NP swab) at a COVID-19 Assessment Centre? The previous testing method provided more accurate data and useful information. Face mask mandates were terminated (except for health care workers) on March 21, 2022. It sounds like we are cutting corners to save money, not to save lives. It also gives protesters and the public the idea the pandemic is over, but nurses and doctors know the truth. Only the emergency phase is over. Check the Public Health Agency of Canada and WHO websites for the best available updates.

As of July 5, 2023, my hospital has made masks optional in most public areas of the building. However, nurses still use masks in patients' rooms. It's true there are fewer COVID-19 cases and deaths, but we're not out of the woods yet.

I'm still unclear as to what Temporary Pandemic Pay was about. At first, I thought it was the provincial government's *mea culpa* for Bill 124. I was optimistic that Premier Ford and his government finally realized their mistake but couldn't undo the wage suppression legislation. To save face, this was their remedy.

The stated goal was to "help frontline staff who are experiencing severe challenges and are at heightened risk during the COVID-19 outbreak." I didn't hear the word "nurses," but I was sure we were included.

However, the definition of frontline was broader than I expected, just like the essential worker. The eligible workplaces were health care, LTC, retirement homes, social services, and corrections (correctional services). In health care public hospitals were included, and that meant me.

The eligible workers in these hospitals were: PSWs, RNs, RPNs, NPs, attendant care workers, auxiliary staff (housekeepers, porters, screeners, etc.), and RTs. No physiotherapists (PTs) or occupational therapists (OTs). I remember they were upset about being excluded, despite how closely they had to interact with patients for their work. Hospitals advocated in May 2020 for all staff to be included, but the government refused to budge.

This benefit was retroactive pay (retro pay) for the period of April 24, 2020 to August 13, 2020. The formula was $4 above hourly wages and an additional $250 for each four-week period. And of course, taxes were deducted as per usual after all this fanfare.

I was not appeased by any means. Again, I say, the government saw the public reacting to frontline workers as health care heroes and warriors, and decided to join in. A case of *#OntarioToo* and not a sign of leadership.

CHAPTER 29

Efforts to Retain Nurses

Then there was Retention Pay for nurses in Ontario. It was called the Temporary Retention Incentive for Nurses program. This time it was specifically for full-time nurses and pro-rated for part-timers and casual nurses. The $5,000 retention bonus was meant to show good faith, and retain hard-working nurses during our crisis.

But it was revealed that it would be delivered in two payments. To receive $2,500, one had to have worked for an eligible employer from March 20, 2022 to April 22, 2022. To get the full amount the nurse had to be still working as of September 1, 2022.

I was not tempted by this carrot. I retired in June 2022. I wasn't going to stay for an extra three months for this. I had started my retirement countdown in 2015. It was a matter of choosing June or December 2022. It was already clear to me that June 2027 (age 65) was pushing things, despite the best pension outcome. The ongoing COVID-19 situation and the new style of electronic charting and scanning barcodes was too much for me. Just thinking of scanning IDs and medications, basically everything, was overwhelming. It would mean less time for actual patient care. That was a big dilemma for me.

Most of the nurses I knew who could retire already did. One new nurse had already left for the US for better wages and a signing bonus. The rest of the nurses felt stuck where they were and had to learn the new online charting system on top of everything else.

First, there has been a nursing shortage my whole nursing career. It is not primarily a generational issue. Second, with the last two union contracts with a capped 1% salary increase during the pandemic (because of Bill 124), I feel it's not nearly enough (re: inflation or cost of living). There are sign-ing bonuses for nurses in the US of $10,000 or more. Third, the provincial government has all this money for pandemic-related incentives but refuses to accept the repeal of Bill 124 and pay us "retro pay" of the last three years. Four, the disrespect for nurses by the province continues.

Premier Ford acknowledged that Bill 124 didn't exist anymore (January 2023), but his government was still working behind the scenes to appeal the coalition of unions' successful repeal of Bill 124 (*CTV News*, November 29, 2022). "Ford government appeals Ontario court decision striking down Bill 124" confirms this (*The Canadian Press*, December 29, 2022).

Meanwhile, the affected workers cheered as "Ontario hospital nurses awarded additional pay after Bill 124 struck down" (Allison Jones, *The Canadian Press*, April 28, 2023). By the way, I did notice the same article was carried by all the news sources. This news was about the arbitrators of the relevant collective agreements, who proceeded as if the appeal of Bill 124 wasn't still in play. I don't expect any of this money soon. Ford's government can still appeal to the Supreme Court of Canada or just use the "notwithstanding clause" to override every decision so far.

"Why Ontario is in court (again) fighting to save Bill 124" (John Michael McGrath, *TVO Today*, June 20, 2023) is not a difficult question for me. The Conservatives believe they can manipulate the law to deliver election promises. The Court of Appeal for Ontario met in June 2023 and no decision has been made yet.

In the media, Ford's government has moved to enable private clinics to alleviate the backlog of patients needing cataract and hip surgeries. Where is he finding these doctors and nurses if there's a shortage? From other provinces or countries? And will OHIP (Ontario Health Insurance Plan) pay for all of it when it has already delisted certain procedures (like eye exams and dental work) and medications? It doesn't sound like a real effort to keep nurses in hospitals.

CHAPTER 30

Federal Support for Lost Jobs

In contrast to the provincial government, I had more respect for the federal government's actions, which didn't affect me at all. At the beginning of the pandemic the federal government rolled out the Canada Emergency Response Benefit (CERB). Prime Minister Trudeau's government understood that COVID-19 was bigger than SARS (or anything else) and needed immediate drastic measures to reduce or prevent anticipated health impacts and financial misery.

CERB was to "provide financial support to employed and self-employed Canadians who were directly affected by COVID-19." It was a "large-scale public policy … to prevent financial distress for as many people as possible" as described by Luc Godbout in his article "CERB: From Emergency To Recovery" in the *Perspectives on Tax Law & Policy*, September 3, 2020.

The program was effective from March 15, 2020 and ended September 27, 2020. Individuals would receive $2,000 for a four-week period ($500/ week). Yes, there were complications and revisions. But overall, those who received CERB were grateful. So grateful that some people didn't look for work right away, and that became another problem.

Meanwhile, health care workers like nurses had to double down their efforts. I recall wishing I too could stay at home and be paid to isolate or be compensated for my lost job. I was envious at times.

However, I would have also been stressed not knowing if my job was waiting for me, or if I had overextended my finances with a mortgage or that last vacation. Would my bills get paid?

According to Bankruptcy Canada (licensed insolvency trustee), national consumer bankruptcies are down for the last few years. In 2020 they went down by 39.57% from the previous year. StatCan confirms this, noting bankruptcies in 2019 were 54,409, in 2020 they were 32,880, and in 2021 they were 27,461. According to Innovation, Science and Economic Development Canada (ISED) in 2022 there were 24,586 consumer bankruptcies—a reduction of 10.5%, while there was an increase in consumer proposals (a different financial animal).

I believe the CERB program made a huge difference. However, other factors and other stressors may have taken priority, such as utility and banks offering deferrals, and lockdowns closing the court system. The article, "Insolvency Statistics: The Impact of COVID-19 Pandemic on Bankruptcy and Consumer Proposal Filings," is an insightful read on the trustee's website (bankruptcy-canada.ca). It suggests "many consumers have yet to come to grips with what has happened …".

Time will tell. Perhaps those at risk will choose to reassess their lifestyle, and cut back to repay their debt. Maybe instead of bankruptcies, more people will choose consumer proposals and those statistics will rise. I do know I chose to downsize in 2020 instead of 2022, as originally planned. I moved to a smaller home in another city and I'm glad I did.

I also know of small business owners who lost their businesses and had to adapt to make money. Some people rose to the challenge of difficult times. There were also self-employed people who no longer had customers for their product or service and had to rethink their financial strategy. Could they wait out the pandemic? How long were people expected to wait? No one knew.

The federal government showed leadership with the CERB program and with direct fund transfers. According to the Department of Finance Canada (December 2022) the feds also gave huge transfers to the provinces and territories for COVID-19 spending. "Approximately eight out of every ten dollars committed to fight COVID-19 and support Canadians was provided by the Liberal federal government." This contributed to the budgetary surpluses of many provinces and territories.

Juxtapose that with the Ontario provincial government, which continues to work against nurses and other unionized public workers, during a pandemic, no less.

Where's the money from the federal transfer? As a hospital nurse I'm waiting for my retro pay from my union contracts from 2020 to 2022. The provincial government will continue to delay reparations as they try to revive Bill 124. The Ontario Court of Appeals heard the government's legal argument June 23, 2023, and no timeline has been given for a decision.

I'm betting Justice Koehnen knew his original decision would be challenged and wrote a sound legal explanation in his 80-page document. The rest of us are holding our collective breath. It's too early to celebrate.

Maybe I'll just get a belated apology or a medal someday. I won't forget or forgive Ontario's political interference anytime soon.

CHAPTER 31

Nurses' Union (ONA)

In Ontario the nurses' union worked flat out during the pandemic. ONA had already taken the initiative to challenge Bill 124 within a month of its existence. They organized rallies, and email campaigns to protest this new slap in the face towards nurses. It was a long journey with other affected unions joining the battle.

Unions matter. We are stronger together. Try negotiating a pay raise *on your own* or complaining about working conditions *on your own*. Some of my fellow nursing colleagues forget this part. They keep repeating that we have a union and pay union dues but have nothing to show for it. They are so wrong and perhaps unaware of what unions are all about.

I grew up knowing unions were good. My father benefitted from the union at CNR. His job was protected as he got better at it. He only had to show up at the strike line once to get his strike pay. Much later my oldest brother was also in a teachers' union and spent some time on the executive board. So, when I had the opportunity to be involved in starting a union at CIBC Mortgage, I was enthusiastic.

It was, however, a tale of two unions at 750 Lawrence Avenue West, Toronto, with two buildings connected by a cafeteria. In the west building was CIBC Mortgage—a small department (maybe 40–100 people). In the east building was CIBC Visa—a bigger department buried in the high security basement (200–300 people). Both unions started at the same time. Wikipedia only describes this in the broadest of strokes.

Being involved in a union, especially a new one, was very hard. It was all volunteer work back then. The CIBC Mortgage union lasted only a year because the employer had misled certain staff to bring down our small union. The employer was successful in converting two key employees to act as company agents and spread disinformation to the union members. One of these two agents confessed afterwards to doing this and heavily regretted it.

Years later all the jobs were relabeled as Clerk 1, Clerk 2, and so on. I was no longer a Mortgage Life Insurance Clerk. We also had to re-apply for our jobs. I had several diehard pro-CIBC Mortgage supporters tell me afterwards how remorseful they were now that we had decertified our union. They felt their company loyalty had been betrayed.

CIBC Visa employees were more vigilant, vocal, and cohesive and remain today members of the United Steelworkers union. These employees had a lot more grievances than we ever had. I remember when they went on strike in 1986.

Hospital nurses in Ontario can't strike due to the Hospital Labour Disputes Arbitration Act of 1990. I don't think anyone who works in a hospital really wants to go on strike. But the ability to strike is usually a union's strongest negotiating tool. That's why negotiation and arbitration of contracts is so vitally important to nurses. We don't have the same leverage as other unions.

Despite that, being in an established union like ONA is such a relief in comparison. They've been in place for 50 years now, and they know a thing or two about employers.

As of 2023 ONA represents 68,000 nurses and health care professionals, and 18,000 nursing students' affiliates. Values promoted are "strength and unity, integrity and professionalism, and diversity, equity and inclusion." These need to be upheld when threatened.

Sitting back and letting ONA do all the work is not enough. As union members nurses need to be aware of their workplace environment and participate whenever they can to make it better. On the job, the simplest action is to fill out a workload report form when patient or employee safety is at risk. The public needs to know the inside story.

These workload report forms look easy to complete, but they are not. Hypothetically, an individual can fill one out, but there's no weight if one employee complains. It's best if all the nurses from that shift sign the form. However, the onus is still on the nurses to have tried to ameliorate the situation first.

My nursing unit filled out two workload report forms that I signed. I was hesitant to sign because I knew nothing would come of it. However, in a show of solidarity, I did sign. All it did was get the manager upset with us. The heavy workloads continued.

In the beginning of my nursing career, we had two PCAs per shift. They helped with peri-care, bed baths, showers, and repositioning and transferring heavy patients. At least a third of neurosurgery and neurology patients are heavy. That means to safely care for these patients requires two staff.

The mix of staff is down to one PCA on the day and evening shift. Nurses must rely on each other or themselves to lift and turn their own patients. Most are busy and unable to respond to a call for assistance. A nurse will try to lift a patient on her/his own. We are mindful that dragging a patient up in bed is frowned upon as it can cause shearing injuries to the patient's buttocks.

I have had many injuries over the years, but some are repetitive due to the nature of our work. I think the first injury to my right elbow (medial epicondylitis) was in 2013. I had two weeks of modified duties, and then physiotherapy for six months.

I reinjured my right elbow in October 2018 and started physio right away. This time I tried to delay letting anyone know at work. My family doctor ordered an X-ray and ultrasound of the elbow and a referral to an orthopedic surgeon. In February 2019 I saw the specialist, who recommended an MRI, and modified duties for two months.

This time Occupational Health wanted a meeting with my manager and me. Thankfully, my union representative was present and provided moral support. I had not lost any time from work, but modified duties were a bureaucratic headache for everyone. Also, there weren't too many options for modified duties on my unit. Being the Charge Nurse was one possibility which I dreaded, and the other was monitoring patients with epilepsy. I was scheduled for a bit of both.

Bless my family doctor, she didn't give up on me when my MRI showed nothing to fix surgically. She sent me for a second opinion, this time to a sports orthopedist. This doctor had me do shockwave therapy at his recommended physiotherapy clinic, and then platelet-rich plasma injection (PRP).

I finally got relief after the PRP treatment in September 2019. However, I was not warned how painful the procedure would be. A little warning would've helped. Pre-medication would've been a better plan. I'm sure a professional athlete would've had this injury treated much sooner than I did.

Although most of the time our patient load was four per nurse, the severity of our patients and the demands of patients and their family members continued to grow in recent years. The pandemic made these things worse. I wish there was a way to measure the stress levels of nurses on the job. I know I had to manage by compartmentalizing my thoughts, feelings, and aches to get through the shift.

When you're stressed you make mistakes. A mistake has the potential to contribute to more mistakes. I sometimes felt like I was a magnet for "difficult" or complicated patients. If it wasn't my turn, it would have been somebody else's turn on the unit.

Nurses need unions in our hospitals. While nurses care about their patients first, someone should care about the nurses and support and/or protect them. We don't need a government devaluing the work of nurses and interfering in our union contracts. ONA cares about hospital nurses like me and will fight for us.

CHAPTER 32

ONA's Response to COVID-19

It is impressive to read ONA's "COVID-19 Chronicles" on their website (ona.org/covid-19-series-advocacy). Their *COVID-19 Timeline* is a brief history of events and the union's actions. Context matters. ONA had just submitted a legal challenge to Bill 124 in December 2019, and then COVID-19 emerged quietly in January 2020.

The two nurses who had died from SARS were also ONA members. When a novel coronavirus emerged in January 2020 the union was very apprehensive. The Ontario Minister of Health's response to the union's queries was "awareness of the situation." Unsatisfied, the ONA CEO Bev Mathers began to review the old SARS files and recommendations, and then started consulting health and safety specialists. ONA members needed to be protected better this time.

Events heated up in March 2020. The first LTC resident died March 8 at Lynn Valley Care Centre in North Vancouver, BC. It was heavily downplayed in the media (no cause for panic here). Then, on March 10, the

Ontario government denied COVID-19 was airborne (based on the best science at the time) and restricted N95 masks. On March 12 (and revised March 30), the Chief Medical Officer of Health of Ontario issued Directive #1 for Health Care Providers and Health Care Entities advising of an immediate risk to health care workers due to COVID-19. Directive #2 on March 19 cancelled all non-essential and elective surgeries. On March 21 the government issued an order on work redeployment in hospitals. Directive #3 on March 22 advised LTC residents to ban short-stay absences. ONA negotiated with the province March 25–28 on N95 mask usage and other PPE. On March 30 COVID-19 Outbreak guidelines for LTC were published.

April 2020 was also a very hectic month. On April 1 there were 100 deaths in Canada, which jumped to 1,000 by April 15. Revised Directive #3 on April 8 stated all staff and visitors in LTC facilities must wear face masks. Then revised Directive #5 on April 10 mandated N95 masks for aerosol generating procedures for all health care workers, including LTC. On April 15 came an Emergency Order limiting work to one LTC site. ONA filed an emergency application in court on April 16 as some LTC facilities were not complying with directives. April 22 saw the military called to Ontario and Québec to help with severely short-staffed LTC sites. By April 28 there would be 50,000 COVID-19 cases nationwide.

In May 2020 ONA started arbitration for LTC for PPE, IPAC, and resident/staff cohorting. By May 12, there were 5,080 deaths and 69,905 cases. Brian Beattie, RN, who worked at Kensington Village in London, ON, is the first ONA member to die of COVID-19. On May 21 a revised Directive #2 allowed limited hospital admissions to restart. ONA requested on May 22 an independent public inquiry into the situation in LTC. On May 26 the "military report reveals extreme neglect and horrific conditions" in five LTC facilities in Ontario. Then, on July 29, a LTC Commission is announced.

On December 14, 2020, the first health care worker, Anita Quidangen, a PSW from The Rekai Centre (LTC) in Toronto, was vaccinated. She was also the first HCW to get her second dose vaccination on January 4, 2021.

By January 11, 2021, Ontario had more than 5,000 deaths, and a surge in hospital admissions. On January 15 ONA tried again to get nurses and other health care workers exempt from Bill 124. ONA wrote an open letter, dated January 25, to Premier Ford requesting recognition of airborne transmission of COVID-19 and the related precautions (i.e., N95 masks). By January 28 there will be more than 6,000 deaths in Ontario.

On February 25, 2021 ONA filed "urgent judicial review" to change Directives to protect HCWs from COVID-19 asymptomatic transmission, not just aerosol generating procedures.

The Canadian Institute for Health Information (CIHI) advises that by January 14, 2022, there were at least 46 HCW deaths related to COVID-19. Of those deaths, 17 were in Ontario. How many of these deaths could have been prevented if N95 masks were used at work from the start?

As we know now, in 2023, there are many infected people without symptoms. We have stopped mask mandates in the community and other precautions like social distancing. Access to PCR testing is limited. The once abundant home kits are on the decline too. However, hospital nurses continue to work extra hard and wear the full PPE on duty. Beneath the protective gear, one can expect foggy glasses and open-mouth breathing. Taking sips of water becomes less frequent. More respect should come with monetary worth. It is so with professional athletes.

Nursing in hospitals is often very physical and easy breathing is required. Lifting, bending, or twisting are some of the job's repetitive actions. I can't do my work if something is sprained and I have pain. Like an athlete, my body is a tool I must use, perhaps not to the same level or for the same goal.

When I hurt my right elbow, I went through several months waiting for tests and referrals before I came across a Sports Medicine doctor, who connected me to a Sports Chiropractor. He's the one who compared nurses to athletes, and gave me the same exercises for my tendons that he suggested to hockey players. I felt acknowledgement and respect. Unions also show respect for their members when they support and fight for us.

CHAPTER 33

The Bill 124 Court Challenge

The court challenge to Bill 124 began September 12, 2022. For the first time I heard, "Long Live the King" in Canada. It was a reminder that Queen Elizabeth had recently died, and a lot of change was imminent for the countries of the Commonwealth.

ONA had provided links to register to view the streamed court proceedings. I already had some experience watching Zoom meetings, which became a very popular form of communication between employers and employees during the pandemic.

I thought it was only ONA presenting. However, more than 40 affected unions had joined the cause. First up was the Ontario Federation of Labour (OFL), Canada's largest labour organization. It is the umbrella group of 54 Ontario unions, representing more than a million workers. ONA presented next. In total, there were 10 applicants against the Crown (or respondent).

I'm not sure how much I can say about the actual proceedings. The judge made comments the following day that some audio recordings and screen shots had been made by viewers and posted them online. Those actions are prohibited, just like photos of the defendant or witnesses in court are forbidden (hence the court artistic drawings you see on TV). I made some notes instead.

I found it fascinating and at times boring. Everyone had technical difficulties at some point. Not all the participants were in the same court room. Some of the applicants (union lawyers) covered the same legal territory but from a new perspective.

Kate Hughes was the counsel for ONA. She reminded everyone how 90% of ONA members do not have the right to strike. And, that 92% of ONA members are female, suggesting gender discrimination in the type of public servants chosen to moderate their wage increases. The excluded categories were mostly male-dominated occupations or industries.

She went on to discuss the optimal staffing ratio for nurses as 70% full-time, and 30% part-time or casual. However, part-time and casual nurses don't have guaranteed hours, and no company benefits or pension plan.

Stripped down to the legal arguments that ONA put forth are Section 2(d) of the Canadian Charter of Rights and Freedoms re: freedom of association clause, and Section 15 re: equality of rights. The first accused the provincial government of substantial interference of our rights to freedom of association and collective bargaining. The second charged violation of the equality of rights.

I had no idea how important the Canadian Charter of Rights and Freedoms would become for me. I remember when it was brought forth by the federal Liberal government led by former PM Pierre Trudeau in 1982. I was more impressed with the repatriation of the BNA Act of 1867, and the new Constitution Act of 1982, which included the Charter. And now I got to see how this charter applied to me.

The applicants' arguments and legal precedents sounded very persuasive. The Crown's counsel was just as confident while twisting the interpretation of the Charter. However, by the end of the proceedings, I couldn't tell who had won.

ONA had union contracts, where the arbitrators agreed they could not negotiate with Bill 124 in existence. Their hands were tied. I had two contracts during this "moderation period." The Stout Award (April 2020–April 2021) and the Gedalof Award (June 2021–March 2023) were contracts where the 1% wage increase was enforced like the edict it was. Arbitrator Stout had been quoted as saying he would've given 1.75% wage increase if not for Bill 124.

Meanwhile, Arbitrator Gedalof had included a "Reopener" clause should Bill 124 be "declared unconstitutional by a court of competent jurisdiction, … or repealed." That happened. Justice Koehnen repealed Bill 124 as of November 29, 2022, based on **substantial interference** of Section 2(d) of the Charter.

Since Bill 124's demise I haven't heard of any goodwill or action for remedies to this very important legal event from the government. Only unrelated entries show up on the government's 7,000 search results (March 2023). Premier Ford admitted Bill 124 doesn't exist (as a sound bite) but has appealed the decision and the appeal's decision is pending (June 2023).

In the past he has been quoted as saying, "health care workers are seriously underpaid" or "I love nurses." Yet, privately, his government has decided to appeal the Koehnen decision (i.e., resuscitate Bill 124). For the moment, my union has gone back to the negotiating table for the next set of union contracts.

Meanwhile, the Financial Accountability Office of Ontario (FAO) revealed, on March 1, 2023, that the provincial government spent $1.2 billion less in the health sector. The previous year, in the article, "Fiscal watchdog finds Ontario spent $7.2 billion less than planned, projects smaller deficit," the FAO was quoted as saying, "If government underspending becomes a trend, it'll be worth a deeper look." (*CBC News*, July 19, 2022).

In April 2023, "ONA was successful in achieving reopener clauses in the collective agreements, allowing the union to seek retroactive wages should the bill be overturned," and it was overturned. (ONA, "Bill 124 Reopener Decisions Not Nearly Enough to Retain, Recruit Nurses and Health-Care Professionals in Ontario," April 28, 2023). Additional wages expected are 0.75% for the 2020 term, 1% for 2021, and 2% for 2022.

Even my hospital has contacted me to ask if I wanted this retro pay. I did receive my Bill 124 retro pay in September 2023, but I remained anxious.

What if I must return it? Ford was still fighting the decision at this point.

However, we are now waiting for the Appeals Court decision. Everyone else has cooperated except for the Ontario government.

CHAPTER 34

Anti-Mandate Protests

The protests I grew up with had a certain structure. You call people or advertise intent to gather to protest a cause. The cause can be anything, but the intent is to gather, speak your mind or wave your signs, maybe march to a government building, and hope for attention by the intended media or government. Then, after 2–3 hours, you leave.

Several protest convoys of truckers (from the western and eastern provinces) came to Ottawa on January 29, 2022, and did not leave. They crossed the line of good behaviour. The crowd got bigger, and the participants acted like college students on an extended winter break down south, like what you see in movies.

These unvaccinated truckers (and later, their families) were illegally vacationing on the streets of Ottawa. They had parties, stole food from a soup kitchen for the homeless, disrespected national statues, honked car horns all day long, enjoyed a hot tub and fireworks, and refused to move when asked. Being polite didn't work.

I have participated in several protests over the years: Freedom for Moroz (an imprisoned Ukrainian nationalist writer), antinuclear weapons, Invasion of Crimea (Ukraine) 2014, and for ONA several times. These were orderly protests and did not block any transportation (unless we had a permit) or commerce.

I hesitate to call the truckers' protest "Freedom Convoy," since it wasn't about my freedom, the freedom of Ottawa citizens, or any freedom guaranteed by the Canadian Charter of Rights and Freedoms. Section 1 of the Charter states: "Charter rights can be limited by law so long as these limits can be shown to be reasonable in a free and democratic society." Charter rights were never meant to be absolute. I don't think these long-haul truckers did their homework before embarking on this ill-conceived "protest" and subsequent occupation.

When I first heard of the reasoning for this protest convoy, it was as a response to the cross-border truckers being told they had to be vaccinated (January 15, 2022). This was a reciprocal vaccine mandate between the US and Canada. I thought this was a stupid protest, and this story had no legs.

I didn't see what this group hoped to achieve. Their own federation of trucker unions (Canadian Trucking Alliance–CTA) said most of their drivers were already vaccinated and the alliance did not support these protesters. CTA issued strong statements on January 22 and January 29, 2022, denying that all these protesters were truckers. Spencer Boersma supports this in his article "Five misconceptions and four truths about Canada's 'Freedom Convoy'" (February 24, 2022, *Baptist News Global*). He wrote, "At the peak of the protests [in Ottawa], there were about 1,100 vehicles in the downtown but only 230 trucks." Makes one wonder who these protesters really were.

Little did I know about the protesters' GoFundMe account, protest organizers and influencers, cross-country border blockades, or several Conservative government sympathizers. I did know, of course, about the Internet celebs like Elon Musk and Donald Trump, who talked trash. Billionaires can afford to get away with a lot, without the same backlash as the rest of us.

The protesters' message changed from being about international long-haul truckers being forced to get vaccinated against COVID-19 to cross our borders. This only affected the remaining 15% of truckers not yet vaccinated during Wave 5 of the pandemic in Canada.

The new protest message was expanded to include all COVID-19 mandates. So why were they still going to Ottawa? Most of the mandates were provincial, so why weren't they at the capital cities of their province like Toronto or Edmonton? Maybe Toronto Mayor John Tory was smart to maintain his city's State of Emergency after all.

As a health care worker I resented these protests and the actions of those involved. First, these protesters objected to being vaccinated due to their jobs (under any circumstance), while being among one of the first designated essential workers during the pandemic. Second, they were potentially spreading the pandemic virus in two countries. Third, later they would hassle people wearing face masks in Ottawa. And fourth, hospitals were still in crisis mode. Two hospitals had called Code Orange earlier in January 2022. It felt like a personal insult when I had to gear up with my hospital PPE to do my job—to protect my patients, my family, and myself from the COVID-19 infection. How dare they claim to be fighting for Canadian freedoms!

• • •

It seems to me the immediate response to these protesters in Ottawa was overly tolerant. Leadership misread them as benign, rather than the potential threat they were, and so began a game of political chess. There were so many major players taking part that chess seems like the wrong comparison, but there were mainly two groups: the convoy protesters with mostly anonymous supporters, and the police services along with several levels of governments.

I used the local Ottawa newspaper as my main reference for the series of events during this excitable time. The *Ottawa Citizen* article, "The occupation of Ottawa: a timeline" written by Andrew Duffy on February 18, 2022, had many details. Ottawa Police Chief Peter Sloly was correct in saying, on January 26, 2022, that the convoy protest was a "very fluid situation."

However, by January 27, 2022, Chief Sloly had made his first mistake. He was told to keep the truckers away from Parliament Hill but didn't. He felt he was dealing with the regular protesters, who came and left after a few hours. I'm sure he has seen many groups of protesters do this in the past.

The same can be said of protesters at Queen's Park in Toronto. But he was wrong. I don't think he was the only one to believe this.

It was already reported on January 24, 2022 that convoys of truckers, several kilometres long, were approaching Ottawa. By January 29 there were about "3,000 trucks and 15,000 protesters" in Ottawa. Then another trucker convoy blockaded the border at Coutts, Alberta on January 30. This was going to be big.

Chief Sloly made his second mistake on January 31, 2022, when he refused to use force to make arrests. The truckers' wives and children had not arrived yet. He couldn't condone his police force to appear to act like our American counterpart, with the potential for misuse of power or violence. I'm thinking of headlines like, "Former Police Officer Found Guilty of Violating an Arrestee's Civil Rights by Using Excessive Force" in West Virginia, reported by the Office of Public Affairs on November 18, 2021.

All the protesters had cellphones capable of streaming live events. Chief Sloly probably thought to give the protesters more time to leave peacefully. Instead, more protesters arrived. Ottawa had ceased to be peaceful since the first day of the arrival of the intimidating convoys.

I know it's a Canadian character flaw and strength that we hope for the best. Persuasion and other communication attempts didn't get anywhere. It was past time to move on and escalate actions.

Ottawa is not a federal municipal entity like Washington, DC in the US. So, when the US Capitol Building in their capital city was attacked by Trump sympathizers on January 6, 2021, it was the Capitol Police who took charge initially, then aided by the National Guard and DC Metropolitan Police. There was no occupation of the streets (as it had been for weeks in Ottawa), but a lot of violence and property damage. By 8:00 p.m. that day the protesters and rioters were arrested. No occupation, but a wounded nation.

Ottawa Mayor Jim Watson and Ottawa Police Chief Peter Sloly were the primary decision makers. Why did the mayor wait until February 6, 2022 to call a State of Emergency? Why weren't there more voices urging different solutions or more resources? Was the strategy just to get more officers, but still not use force? To intimidate the occupiers with only a greater number of officers? I think everyone was intimidated by the big Mack trucks.

On February 3, 2022 protest organizer Tamara Lich told the media *they plan to stay*. The gauntlet was thrown. Who picked it up but a young woman named Zexi Li, a data analyst, who started a class action lawsuit against the organizers on February 4. Later, this lawsuit would be expanded to include the Ottawa residents and business owners. Now the lawsuit has 15,000 claimants. At the time, the police tried a "surge and contain" strategy to improve safety. This soft approach on truckers failed. Too little, too late.

Where was the premier of Ontario during this? What was Doug Ford doing? His strategy was to wait and see. I think he was waiting for the federal government to jump in. He was hoping to be re-elected in June 2022 and didn't want to alienate the far-right voters from his Conservative provincial party.

Other conservative party members openly supported the protesters. MPP Randy Hillier made this very inflammatory statement on February 5, 2022: "this is the hill we die on." On February 10, 2022 MP Pierre Poilievre (now federal Conservative opposition leader) stated he stood with the protesters too. These politicians were subverting law and good order.

Meanwhile, MP John Brassard wrote how the Conservatives gave Canadians the Canadian Bill of Rights (1960) in his 2022 Barrie–Innisfil community flyer. There was no reason to mention this in reviewing his and his party's accomplishments for the prior year, other than as a subtle nod to the convoy protesters. Plus, if the Bill of Rights was so great, why did the Liberals have to entrench a better version in the Canadian Charter of Rights and Freedoms, which is part of the Constitution Act of 1982?

It is noteworthy that seven out of ten provinces have Conservative governments, while only one province and one out of three territories are Liberal. Partisan politics were unequivocally a factor in how things got resolved and ultimately perceived. More recently, Alberta Premier Danielle Smith had given moral support to a Coutts border blockade protester by personally calling him (*Global News*, March 29, 2023).

The federal government was, of course, monitoring the situation and staying in its lane. By February 5, 2022, the GoFundMe fund was closed as the government claimed the terms of service were violated. The fundraiser had collected $10 million, then the money had to be refunded. Some of the donors were very suspicious.

I am sure the American government was watching closely as well. On February 7, 2022, the Windsor border was blocked by trucks and protesters on the Ambassador Bridge. This was the busiest Canada–US border crossing. Then, on February 8, another fundraiser, GiveSendGo, this time in the US, raised $6.3 million.

The Ontario government froze the new fundraiser on February 10, 2022. Two weeks after the convoy occupation of Ottawa, on February 11, Ford's provincial government finally declared a State of Emergency to remove the protesters. By February 12 the Ottawa police, OPP, and RCMP were working together, while an influx of weekend protesters showed up.

Premier Ford's motto should be *Open for Convoy Protesters*, not *Open for Business*. Ottawa's businesses lost money during the occupation as did the auto industry from the border blockade. Ford was waiting until the last possible moment to act. I don't see why he hesitated when he had declared so many States of Emergency before. This must have been partisan politics. He wanted the Liberal federal government to make a huge political mistake. The knives were out and ready.

On February 14, 2022 the federal government invoked the Emergencies Act. I say it should have happened sooner, but others feel it should never have been used at all. They probably think the Act is a last resort when it comes to violence. I disagree.

Violence is not the only crime in the Criminal Code of Canada. It would be light reading indeed. It doesn't take a war to cripple a nation. Other crimes can have far-reaching consequences for our independence and nationhood. Blocking trade or transportation is illegal, but using children as shields was unforgivable. The truckers brought their wives and children later to signal they were staying.

Ottawa was occupied by anarchists, not members of a democracy. Did any of these people vote in the last election? Did any of these protesters even realize most of the COVID-19 mandates were provincially regulated, not federally? Were they stupid or misinformed? I don't believe it was heavy-handed to liberate Canada's capital city from their occupation. This was an attack on the symbolic heart of our nation.

Was it just 2017 when we celebrated our country's 150th birthday? I visited Ottawa after the crowds had left. I could still sense the good energy generated. I felt patriotic and signed up to get one of the actual parliament flags. And now this act of civil disobedience has left an open wound. We have gone from love fest to "hate fest" in five years, disrespecting our PM and other Canadians. Canadians who got vaccinated and still follow provincial mandates or wear face masks for protection.

The Emergencies Act was also used to liberate our border crossings with the US. How long do you think the US would tolerate disruption of their economic trade? NAFTA was at risk. How embarrassing would it be to have the Americans come to rescue us from other Canadians? Or worse, if the Americans chose to join or replace the occupation? This was a real threat to the security of Canada.

I wish I had heard the conversations between Prime Minister Justin Trudeau and US President Joe Biden, or Deputy PM and Minister of Finance Chrystia Freeland with US Senior Economic Advisor Brian Deese. I'm sure some of the testimony was redacted. It was estimated $6 billion in economic loss due to the week-long closure of the Ambassador border crossing. We could not afford to appear weak or lose our international reputation. The time for tolerance had long passed.

Despite being summoned to appear at the Emergencies Act Inquiry Premier Ford refused to attend, citing parliamentary privilege. I guess he was too busy to reveal how his lack of action escalated tensions, which led to the federal government's final chess move. He can deny as much as he wants, but the premier's absence was deliberately crafted.

The inquiry concluded November 2022. The main questions were whether Trudeau's federal government met the threshold required to use the Act, and if these extraordinary powers were used responsively. I declare they did. Commissioner Paul Rouleau's final report agreed February 17, 2023.

• • •

"Je me souviens aussi." I was frightened for my country during the occupation of Ottawa and the border blockades. The last time I felt this way was in 1980 when the province of Québec was threatening to separate and had its first referendum. I could not imagine a Canada without Québec, and I became a scared teenager. What was Canada without Québec?

In 1980 the people of Québec voted 60% not to separate from Canada. Then the next referendum was even more shocking. *In 1995 only 51% voted no.* This was too close for comfort. What would happen to ship travel on the St. Lawrence River? Would the region of Ungava be reclaimed and given to Nunavut or Newfoundland and Labrador? This gave me heart palpitations just thinking about it. Instead of separation the province isolated itself even more with its French-only signage.

In grade five I had been on a student exchange trip to Sherbrooke, Québec. It was fun, and Caroline's family went out of their way to make me feel comfortable despite my poor French. That was a great week.

We had only started learning French the year before in school. However, I didn't realize we were taught Parisian French, not Québécois French. Maybe if the Ontario school boards changed this we'd get along better with our neighbouring province.

Whenever I saw the Québec licence plate, *Je me souviens*, I thought it referred to the referendum and I would get upset again. It used to be *La belle province* but changed in 1978 to the current one—two years before the referendum. However, I recently discovered this phrase was an old motto from the 1883 coat of arms of the Québec provincial parliament. It's a reference to Samuel de Champlain's arrival in North America in 1603.

I certainly wish more people knew this. I also want to reiterate Québec (Lower Canada) joined Ontario (Upper Canada), New Brunswick, and Nova Scotia in a union in 1867. Not as the defeated French colony of 1763. So, Québec wanting to separate is more like a unilateral divorce. I hope we have given our fellow Canadians enough space and freedom to stay in our confederation.

But alas it seems Québec is still restless. Jillian Page writing in the *Montreal Gazette*, "Les Québécois: Conquered, but not assimilated" (2014) suggests the "sovereignty dream is very much alive." And my anxiety peaks again. I feel hopeless because Québec still wants to be a separate nation despite the good-will of other Canadians. It may be their dream, but it is my nightmare.

During the pandemic, Ontario and Québec were at times neck in neck with the highest COVID-19 case counts. Ontario has a population of 15 million (2023), but Québec has half of that. Each province and territory managed this health care crisis their own way. Since the pandemic is not over yet, one cannot judge whose management was best.

Meanwhile, the eastern provinces decided to reduce the virus spread with *Atlantic Bubble* travel restrictions originally July 3, 2020–November 26, 2020, and a few times after that. I had only recently heard of this successful strategy. However, this did not stop truckers from the Atlantic provinces joining the convoys to Ottawa.

Other convoys went to block border crossings. They figuratively sat on the line (the borders) and reveled in it. Both protester groups had big Mack trucks. Don't tell me this wasn't organized, or that I had nothing to fear.

• • •

Valentine's Day 2022 was the beginning of the end of Ottawa's occupation. On February 15, 2022, Ottawa Police Chief Peter Sloly resigned and was replaced by Interim Chief Steve Bell. The Coutts border blockade ended, and a cache of firearms and ammunition was found. Thirteen people were arrested.

On February 17, 2022 the police start arresting protesters in Ottawa after warning them the day before. Protest organizers Tamara Lich and Chris Barber were arrested. The downtown restaurant owners of Ottawa joined Zexi Li's class action suit and increased the damages sought from the initial $9.8 million to $306 million.

By February 18, 2022 the initially hesitant tow truck drivers had now removed the trucks left behind. I guess the Emergencies Act made them more compliant. Pat King, a COVID-19 conspiracist and spreader of disinformation, was arrested and charged with perjury and obstruction of justice, amid other lesser charges. On that day the police arrested 70 people and towed 21 vehicles, according to Duffy's article.

Between February 17 and February 20, 2022 protesters and vehicles were removed, and blockades were dismantled. The 23 days of Ottawa's occupation was over. Our national borders were open for trade and transportation.

The Emergencies Act was revoked after nine days on February 23, 2022. It's a good thing too, because the very next day Russia invaded Ukraine. Canada is in a much stronger position internationally now than if we had not resolved our domestic impasse. We are not weaklings or doormats. I hope we continue to choose our fights carefully.

•••

It's hard to go out and protest the "anti-vaxxers" or the anti-COVID-19 mandate protesters when you are busy working in the hospital during a pandemic. I know I was exhausted. Therefore, I really appreciate all the Canadians who did this on our behalf.

These are the counter protests that I'm aware of. On February 5, 2022 there were "convoy resistance" protests in Ottawa, Vancouver, and Whitehorse. On February 12 Toronto was scheduled for one too, but it was cancelled due to the new Ontario State of Emergency declared the day before.

I remember trying to get to Toronto General Hospital for some appointment during this time. University Avenue was closed at College Street. I had heard news that employees had some difficulty getting into the hospital due to anti-COVID mandate protesters. I knew about the planned counter protest and hoped to attend, but I was going to be working that day. I didn't know it was cancelled.

On February 13, 2022 Ottawa residents blocked new convoy arrivals from joining the entrenched group. I'm glad the residents were not defeated and took what action they could. Perhaps the local police should have thought of doing this or deputized the residents.

Unfortunately, in July 2023 there is still an anti-mandate and anti-vaccine lingering presence. Maybe it's now morphed into an anti-Trudeau sentiment? Since the Ottawa occupation, I still see a few people driving cars or trucks with one or two Canadian flags. And it's not about supporting your sports team. It angers me that these protesters have usurped the symbol of being Canadian (our flag) to promote anarchy and selfishness. I see more of these vehicles here in Barrie, than in Newmarket or Toronto.

One more shout out to nurses. On January 28, 2022, the *Toronto Star* had this article: "If truckers were women, no one would care. Just ask nurses." It is strange that professionals who care for others are not themselves cared for, nor supported by others in our community. Penny Mamais writes how millions of dollars were raised for truckers, but no support for nurses. The same nurses "working tirelessly to combat this virus and save lives, while at the same time risking their own."

She goes on to write it's a gender bias. People "throwing money at a group of men—over 96 per cent of truck drivers are male—who do not agree with the vaccine mandate."

Why are Canadians more supportive of truckers than of health care workers? Gender inequality—it's pervasive (UN Women, 2010). Bill 124 turned out to be the same because they deliberately excluded male-dominated sectors. Both nurses and teachers have fewer male workers. The Ontario College of Teachers' 2020 Annual Report reveals gender ratio to be 75% female teachers versus 25% male teachers (https://reports.oct.ca/2020/Statistics/Membership-Demographics). Meanwhile, the statistic for nurses is 91% female to 9% male (as previously stated in Chapter 28). There is an obvious gender gap in these professions, which contributes to the continued gender inequality in the professions.

I am not part of the social media culture, but I believe it's easier than ever to send money to a cause that reflects your concerns, opinions, or community. It's easy to get caught up in rhetoric (e.g., Donald Trump) as balanced reporting seems sparce and elusive among the Internet chatter. Nurses are not looking for charity, but competitive wages that reflect the value they provide for our community.

• • •

If only we could all escape to Mars? I'm sure nurses in a Mars colony would get more respect than they currently do in Ontario. In April 2023 I discovered TALK's (Nick Durocher's) song about Mars. In the article "How The Song Happened: TALK's Run Away to Mars," TALK was inspired and had written the song in March 2020 during Ottawa's lockdown (Howard Druckman, June 26, 2023, socanmagazine.ca). He admitted it was about loneliness and the pandemic. Was the universe listening to his lament and brought the noisy protesters to his town two years later as his music spread on YouTube (first version of the music video, June 2021)? Food for thought. Regardless, it is a very soulful song that is worthy of being an earworm.

Upon further reflection, I think the song's lyrics about running out of oxygen resonate the most with me. While wearing my PPE mask and face shield I admit I felt mild breathlessness. It may have been just a psychological effect of wearing two layers of protection and realizing my mouth was hanging open beneath the mask. While I know there's no study supporting this, I think the humidity of exhaling and rebreathing some of the exhalation caused my discomfort. Alas, I would not make a good astronaut or an immigrant to Mars.

The federal government brought back peace and good order to the capital of Canada. Or as the Constitution Act (1867) states "peace, order and good government" was restored. Protests are allowed in a democratic society. In fact, discourse is encouraged. Intimidation and misinformation are not. However, different points of view enrich our society as it grows and adapts to new circumstances. Escaping the pandemic wasn't an option, but I understand the sentiment. After all, I did run away to Barrie.

Epilogue

A lesson learned from COVID-19 should be the need to recommit to the health of our communities. Rebuilding our Canadian health care system requires renewed commitment to prevention. Everyone wins by preventing disease and infection. It also requires everyone to participate.

I believe every one of us has a duty to our community to be good citizens and care about each other's health. Like companies that show corporate social responsibility (CSR), people should have *community social responsibility*. That includes volunteering time, giving to a worthy cause, donating blood, or signing up for organ donation. In the context of COVID-19, that means doing a personal risk assessment before interacting with other people.

Screening yourself minutes before entering a hospital, business, or group event is not enough. It is way too late. One should assess one's health before leaving the front door. "How are you?" takes on a new value-laden meaning. Switch it around to **How am I today? How am I feeling?** Can you really say to yourself, "I'm fine," and believe it? Remember quality of life has no meaning without your good health.

I recall the 1970s being labelled the Me Decade. I thought that was also the Me Generation. I didn't get it. However, I think the last decade is evidenced by self-absorption and entitlement. Maybe this is due to helicopter parents who didn't get enough as children themselves. Everyone needs to travel, be online to connect to social media, or have the latest iPhone or android cell. Where is the social consciousness in real life? Why is wearing a face mask an oddity in public during a pandemic in Ontario or Canada?

I suggest being a good community citizen starts with *health promotion and respiratory illness prevention*. Currently it means doing a personal risk assessment for contracting COVID-19. Do I need to do a home COVID-19 rapid test before I go out? Do I need to wear a mask to the elevator in my condo or am I relatively safe to get to my car? Do I need to wear a face mask to get a coffee at Tim Hortons or Starbucks? Why do I need a sign stipulating a Mask-Friendly Environment to feel welcomed? The last one is rhetorical.

It depends on whether I have any symptoms or am going to a crowded indoor environment. Depends on the time of day and expected traffic in the elevator. And it depends on if I'm going inside Tim Hortons or using a drive-thru. I guess the biggest concern is **whether, in hindsight, I would be upset that I didn't wear a face mask and either contracted COVID-19 or had spread it to someone else.** That should be our litmus test. We are playing with other people's lives as well as our own.

Some would say just get the COVID-19 infection on purpose to achieve natural immunity. However, natural immunity hasn't been proven to be the safest bet. It's a gamble. Anything can happen once you get infected. New COVID-19 variants are unpredictable. And hybrid immunity, which involves having been fully vaccinated and still getting infected, has not been touted as the best remedy either, only better than no immunity. Don't forget the possibility of *Long COVID syndrome*, the constellation of chronic symptoms of the post COVID-19 infection.

The Government of Canada's website officially calls Long COVID "Post COVID-19 condition." Both adults and children can suffer from it, but symptoms vary between the two groups. For adults, common symptoms are fatigue, trouble sleeping, shortness of breath, general pain and discomfort, cognitive problems, and mental health issues. For children, it's fatigue, headaches, abdominal pain, sleep problems, shortness of breath, cognitive problems, muscle aches, and joint pains.

There are many reasons a smart person would avoid infection.

Wearing a face mask should not be just a personal choice, but a *thoughtful decision* after assessing your risk level and planned activities. The message from our provincial government should be that wearing a mask protects your local community and you. You are not an island. Masking is not a hardship for most when used for short periods of time. As a hospital nurse, I should know.

It seems awkward now to even ask acquaintances or strangers if they've been vaccinated. Even if they have been, that's no guarantee they are not contagious with some respiratory infection during the flu season or another COVID wave. That's why we need Public Health to keep us informed. It should not be so hard to search Ontario's government website to find this data. Transparency and accessibility of government data should go hand in hand. It's in the public's interest to know.

To wear a mask during a pandemic shows you care about your family and community. It may also mean you have symptoms but can't stay at home to isolate yourself. Leaders should be role models for community-desired behaviour. Leaders should not give up, be in denial, or distract us with a new highway in our protected greenspace. COVID-19 is still in our province and in our local community. The WHO reaffirmed COVID-19 is still a pandemic (January 2023) but it's no longer in the emergency phase (May 2023).

It seems some politicians lead by checking the polls for the mood of the people. That's not leadership or science. Sounds instead like you're getting ready to be re-elected. To lead, you need to adapt and pull the community together towards safety and better health. Why haven't we seen more public service announcements (PSAs) to encourage vaccination, or the next booster shot?

All governments have moved from accurate testing and reporting. Resources have moved to other priorities. You now need to qualify to get a PCR test for COVID-19. Websites show "percent positivity" of allowable tests. Wastewater surveillances (WWS) give an estimate of the disease in only 75% of communities in Ontario. Neither indicator should be used to reliably estimate cases. We need to find our own truth.

I am calling on all Canadians to change your behaviours to protect our communities, and our country. Become the role model you want to see. It starts with you caring more about others. Ironically this means keeping yourself healthy too.

I grew up believing we were a caring nation, accepting of immigrants and refugees. Where health care is free and transferable anywhere in Canada. (And where it is not portable, it has to do with the inter-provincial relationships, not the federal government). Health care remains a primary Canadian value. It can improve the quality of life for all of us if only we cared enough about each other.

I was inspired by the phrase "civic responsibility and empathy" expressed by Dr. Nili Kaplan-Myrth on an episode of *The Agenda* with Steve Paikin on TVO. I believe civic duty and empathy for the vulnerable and disadvantaged is never out of fashion. In fact, *being a helpful member of the community* is one of the responsibilities of new (and existing) Canadian citizens.

As Canadians we check the weather before heading out. I'm asking you to go beyond your internal weather check, which may be a mental health assessment for some. Just as we try to avoid inflicting our pain or anger on others, we should avoid inflicting COVID-19 on others.

Ideally, the behaviours I want to see include a daily personal risk assessment of COVID-19 vulnerability outside of your home. Continue to wash your hands properly and frequently. Cough or sneeze into your elbow, not into your hand. Mask in public when there is risk. This means inside businesses, facilities, or in crowded indoor or outdoor gatherings. And know if it is time to get a booster shot.

A side note about community masking. Everyone noticed when Dr. Theresa Tam, Chief Public Health Officer of Canada, hesitated to promote face coverings for the public at the beginning of the COVID-19 pandemic. Eventually she bowed to political or public pressure to recommend it as a tool of prevention against COVID-19 in the community. Her words were, "as another layer of protection" indeed.

I have ruminated over fabric masks for quite some time. I even bought many colourful face masks to wear outside of the hospital. It was fun being creative and making people smile. The animal face masks for adults were the best. But it dawned on me that photos of masked Chinese in the news only showed the blue face masks. Was this because they make them in China or because they're better than cloth face coverings?

I think the political thinking was to leave the blue masks and N95 masks for health care workers as mask shortages had occurred, and to let the public use anything else. There are now enough blue masks and I feel like I should be using one in public.

However, our blue masks are not environmentally friendly. Whatever environmental gains we make by reducing plastics, like plastic straws, the blue masks will have taken up their spot in the landfill. Couldn't we burn garbage like Japan does? Hasn't the technology caught up yet for it to be safe?

The fabric masks (non-medical masks) can be washed and reused. The WHO recommends three-layer fabric masks. But who really washes their fabric mask at the end of the day? Feels like a dilemma.

However, I have recently changed my mind. I went to a family gathering and wore a fabric mask, but removed it for five minutes to eat a slice of cake while distancing myself from others. Over the next few days I had an uncommon cold. I tested myself for COVID-19 several times. Negative results. However, this experience has shown me that if I can catch a cold with this fabric mask, then it does nothing to protect me at all. Better to stick to the blue three-layer procedure masks.

Other recommended behaviours include continuing to social distance two metres (six feet) or one metre (three feet). People have stopped doing this. Improve your own ventilation at home by opening your windows daily for at least 15 minutes. I prefer half an hour. This helps prevent exposure to fine aerosol particles indoors and refreshes your indoor air. Smell the difference afterwards. Inspect your furnace and dryer filters monthly for cleaning or changing. Be aware if ventilation is poor or of unknown quality when you're going to be indoors, then wear a mask (e.g., on an airplane, bus, or train).

I found this phrase, "hands, face, space, ventilate and isolate" in Ian Colbeck's article, "COVID-19: it's freezing outside, but you still need to open your windows," published online February 2021 in *The Conversation*. Even Florence Nightingale wrote about opening windows for the health of her patients in her book, *Notes on Nursing* (1859). The importance of ventilation cannot be overemphasized.

Get tested if symptomatic, or if going to a social event, get tested beforehand. Use your home kit while it's still available. It is better to know you did not infect anyone. Lastly, get vaccinated as many times as it takes. I'm on dose number 5 now.

I'd also revise the previous slogan to "**hands, face, space, ventilate, isolate and vaccinate.**" Doesn't have the same rhythm, but it is an important message that Public Health should spend more time on. Vaccination includes getting available boosters as well. Ontario only has 83.4% fully vaccinated people with two doses as of Jan 12, 2023. I don't think that's enough. There is no magic percentage. It may come down to keeping up with our booster shots. I know we all can do better.

Vaccine hesitancy is a concept I will never understand. Some people would rather listen to influencers like Trump, or other bloggers, or other sources of misinformation and disinformation. Get your medical information about COVID-19 or any health concern from your family doctor, or a recognized medical source like Public Health Ontario or the Public Health Agency of Canada, the CDC, or the WHO.

Vaccines were built on prior vaccine research. Recent data suggest that the mRNA vaccines are better than non-mRNA like the ones China was using. It's true there is no cure for the common cold, but it has been studied. A vaccine for the common cold would be not useful as the symptoms are not life threatening.

That is not the case with COVID-19. Its virus causes severe illness, post-infection syndromes, and death. We know about the virus' variants of concern like Alpha, Beta, Delta, Gamma, and Omicron, and more recently *variants of interest* like XBB.1.5 (Kraken).

Vaccines promise to reduce the severity of the consequences of the COVID-19 infection, which are: being hospitalized for pneumonia, myocarditis, long-term health problems, and death.

In Canada the two main COVID-19 vaccines use mRNA to trigger an immune response to produce antibodies. This technology has been studied, used for some time, and approved for use by Health Canada.

For the very rare severe side effects of the vaccine there is help. To qualify one must provide medical records proving "serious and permanent injury connected to a vaccine authorized by Health Canada."

As of August 11, 2023 Canada has administered 98,439,920 vaccine doses (health-infobase.canada.ca/covid-19/vaccine-administration). Out of this amount, 1,859 claims have been made to the Vaccine Injury Support Program since June 1, 2021 (vaccineinjurysupport.ca/en/program-statistics). This amounts to 0.0019% possibility of having a serious medical side effect from the vaccines. So far, only 103 claims have been approved and settled. Vaccines are certainly worth this negligible risk. I acknowledge this is cold comfort to those who have won the wrong kind of lottery.

Canada is, however, taking care of its citizens, but are the citizens taking care of Canada? No. We should have had a higher percentage of vaccinated people. As of June 18, 2023, only 80.5% of the whole population has been fully vaccinated (had two doses). Newfoundland and Labrador achieved 91.8%, so it is possible (health-infobase.canada.ca/covid-19/vaccination-coverage).

I have seen a wide range of attitudes from laissez-faire to paranoia in the early part of the pandemic. Labourers who don't ask about masking inside your home and believe the previous pandemic mandates were an overreaction. Neighbours who continued with social gatherings in their small space. Then there were those who had asked for their delivered hot food to be left outside on the porch. (It's the norm now but it used to be hand delivered). Or the shopper who wore a chemical respirator with filtered side ports (as seen on disaster movies). I don't believe I'm extreme, but I worked as a bedside nurse during COVID-19. My perspective will be different than yours.

Governments and other institutions have geared down on COVID-19 information. The Ontario Dashboard closed September 8, 2022. Johns Hopkins University stopped collecting COVID-19 data March 10, 2023. The WHO is still monitoring but admits a decrease in member countries providing statistics. This means that a true picture of the situation is inaccurate if cases are being underreported. Therefore, we as individuals must do better on our own and as a community.

I recently heard a doctor from the Peterborough Health Unit describing their community risk assessment. I checked and my regional public health unit in Barrie, Simcoe Muskoka District Health Unit, also has a COVID-19 Community Risk Level site. It includes many of the things I'm promoting, including *a daily personal and situational risk assessment.*

They also have a COVID-19 Community Risk webpage showing simple graphics where we are with five indicators. The data is two weeks behind when community risk level was moderate (April 8, 2023). The trend is decreasing, but the wastewater signal was increasing. Confusing, right? At least I'm not alone in this personal risk assessment concept.

I recall, in the 1990s, the environmental movement called true believers "deep green environmentalists." Perhaps the prevention of COVID-19 needs a citizens' movement and paired colour, too. Maybe blue for the shortness of breath and severe pneumonia of COVID-19, and Long COVID symptoms that linger. I don't mind being known as a "deep blue advocate" for the prevention of COVID-19. "Deep blue preventionist" just doesn't have the same ring to it.

Be COVID Smart. We need to assess the need to take preventive measures before walking out the front door. Reduce your in-person contacts and/or wear a face mask when outside your home. Keep up to date with your vaccines and boosters. COVID-19 is here to stay, and it remains to be seen whether it continues to exist as a pandemic. The disease may become endemic to a region, as with Lyme disease. Do not be complacent. *Know your risk, lower your risk.* Your life or someone else's life may depend on it.

I feel the pandemic has transformed all of us. Escaping to the Moon or Mars is not an option. I have moved on from being a public hospital nurse who assessed patients to being a private citizen who now assesses herself to protect herself and her community. I even considered going back to nursing part-time, but had to update my CPR first.

My last CPR recertification class was in January 2022 at The Michener Institute in Toronto. I was undecided on returning to nursing in 2023 as the need was still great for additional nurses. The course was several hours, and everyone wore a face mask. We all had individual half mannequins, and space between each person. I had let my certification lapse in 2023 and had to take the regular CPR course, so I included first aid at the local CPR provider instead.

My COVID status changed in May 2023. I wore a mask to the first aid and CPR class. No one else did, and so I took it off in the lobby where the instructor was doing attendance. It was a combination of embarrassment and perceived peer pressure. I rationalized that the room was large, had high ceilings, and good ventilation. On the second day of class the instructor said we could have worn a mask. A bit too late. Practising CPR in groups of three people over a mannequin was another mistake. I was sick the following day. It was not worth becoming a member of the hybrid immunity group. I blame myself for not following my own principles. And sadly, I also see this as another sign from the universe. Nursing is now over for me.

I felt I had avoided getting infected by surfing the COVID waves by wearing the hospital's PPE. But once I retired, I succumbed to the virus. I couldn't outrun it anymore. But I believed I could. I wanted so much to be that COVID unicorn.

When I became a "civilian" upon retirement, the rules of prevention were less clear and no longer enforced. I exposed myself to the virus in a moment of hesitancy. To wear a mask, or not wear a mask: that was my question. I failed to head my own advice. I deserved the consequences.

Know yourself. Assess yourself. Know your COVID-19 risk level, today and every day. It may not be COVID-19 next time, but something else.

It's never too late to become *COVID Smart*. What is the alternative—COVID dumb, COVID blind, or worse, mass forgetfulness? There is a current trend of pandemic amnesia, which deliberately ignores that there ever was a respiratory pandemic. This is troubling. Sure, life continues, but hopefully, with the awareness to change our behaviours and habits. The pandemic's almost 7 million deaths (WHO, August 6, 2023), in the context of the information technology era, should matter and should not be forgotten so easily. I know I won't forget because I wrote it down. I invite others to do the same.

The End

Acknowledgements

It is with much gratitude I recognize the contributions and/or collaborations with Maria Scala for premium editing and Laura Boyle for the exquisite cover. Any editing errors are mine from tweaking the final draft. Thanks to Laura Joy for capturing a spark of my personality in her photos. And finally, appreciation for the existence of the Barrie Writers' Club and the suggestions of Marilyn, Bruce, Becca and Nicole.

About The Author

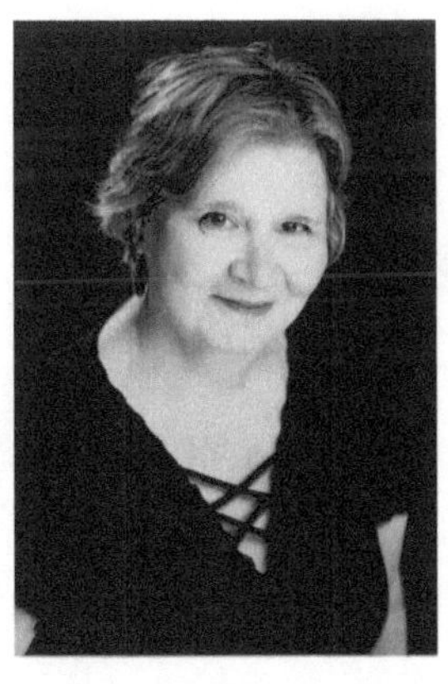

Zenia Kahan is a new writer in the niche world of COVID literature. After almost 20 years of bedside nursing, she has the perspective to comment on the responses to the pandemic of healthcare stakeholders and other groups. She also felt compelled to write about the true work of hospital nurses to reveal misconceptions the public may still have.

Born in Toronto, Canada as the youngest of five children to immigrant parents. She has always explored her environment and later travelled to all seven continents. It is only now she has the time to continue her quest to see the rest of Canada up close and personal. She resides in Barrie, Ontario.

You may reach the author at zkahan.author@gmail.com.